0

Pharmacology:

The Guide to Residency

First edition

(This book is a reproduction of the original book "Internal medicine: The Guide to Residency" to include all the Pharmacology topics with some additions)

Amer Sayed, MD
Georgia Regents University
Internal Medicine Resident

1

DISCLAIMER

Care has been taken to confirm the accuracy of the information presented in this book by reviewing the literature and books related to the subjects and by including the most common practice information and experience from the authors and editors stand of point . However, the authors, editors, and publisher are NOT responsible for errors or omissions or for any consequences from application of the information in this book and make no warranty, expressed or implied, with respect to the currency, completeness, or accuracy of the contents of the publication. Practitioners are responsible for applying this information into patient's care and the clinical out-come

The authors and editors listed the most common medicine and some of the doses used in practice according to their best knowledge, however, it is highly recommended to recheck the medicine indications and doses from an up-to-date source as they change with time. This is particularly important when the recommended agent is a new or infrequently employed drug. And it is the responsibility of the health care provider to ascertain the FDA status of each drug or device planned for use in clinical practice.

**Contact the author by email:
internalmedicinetheguide@gmail.com**

Table of Contents

CONTRIBUTORS

All are from Georgia Regents University

Contributing Authors:
All are Georgia Regents University Residents &
contributed in the following chapters

Eduard Fatakhov, MD
Haytham Alkhaimy, MD
Scott Graupner, MD
Abhishek Mangaonkar, MD
Gita Mehta, MD
Sasha Baker, MD

Contributing Editors:
Lee A Merchen, MD, FACP
Program Director, Internal Medicine Residency

James Gossage, MD
Division of Pulmonary/Critical Care
Professor of Medicine

Pascha Schafer, MD
Divison of Cardiology
Associate Program Director

Lu Huber, MD
Division of Nephrology
Assistant Professor

Gyanendra Sharma, MD, FASE, FACC
Division of Cardiology
Professor of Medicine

Thaddeus Carson, MD
Division of Internal Medicine
Assistant Professor

Meshia Wallace, MD
Internal Medicine Resident

Christina DeRemer, Pharm.D., BCPS
Pharmacy Supervisor, Clinical Service (Medicine)

Mike Garcia, PhD
Director of College Composition
Assistant Professor

Medical Students:
Danielle Bayer
Brandon Taylor
Evan Fountain
Amir Makhmalbaf
Zachary Hoffmann
Reshma Reddy
Kunal Patel
Nader Aboujamous

Medical Illustrator
Michael A. Jensen, MS, CMI
Assistant Professor

Special Acknowledgement
Walter J. Moore, MD, MACP, FACR
Division of Rheumatology
Professor of Medicine and Pediatrics

All GRU staff who provided assistance in this project

Preface

This guidebook is written to assist in the transition between medical school and internal medicine residency; it is designed to highlight the most common clinical cases presented and how best to manage them. The topics have been carefully chosen to cover common differential diagnoses to common symptoms. This book will give you a quick summary of what you need clinically to know about them as well as challenges you may encounter in the process. Ideally, this handbook can be read in 1-2 weeks and consulted at any time during residency, but especially during internship.

By reading this guide, written by current internal medicine residents, the reader will benefit from residents' actual experiences, both successes and missteps, which can aid the reader with patient care and case management. The guide includes managing the common clinical problems that patients are admitted for so the intern or the resident will feel confident and display more accuracy in examining the patient, obtaining medical history, writing a thorough and useful history and physical with appropriate work-up.

Unlike the other few available guide or pocket books, this one will NOT address unnecessary and hard-to-remember details you may NOT need in day-to-day practice in order to deliver the most high-yield information in short period of time. Since fourth-year medical students may have only one to two months of internal medicine training, they may become less familiar in managing common diseases after months of training in other specialties (NOT to mention the time traveling during match season and relocation takes). This book will prove to be efficient and effective even during this busy time.

The focus of this guide will be the common explanations for chest pain like acute coronary syndrome, pulmonary embolism; hyper/ hyponatremia, lower/ upper GI bleed, different types of pneumonia, atrial fibrillation, CHF, and so on. The primary resources and references we have used include *Harrison's Principles of Internal Medicine*, the *Washington Manual of Medical Therapeutics*, several published articles on internal medicine, and other resources. This book offers years of experience from residents and attendings, keeping you, a recent medical graduate, in mind. I must reiterate that the input of the attendings who took time to be a part of this project was crucial. This finished guidebook is a culmination of real clinical experience you will encounter presented in an easy-to-reference format written by the fresh perspective and experience of your fellow internal medicine residents.

Amer Sayed, M.D.
Internal Medicine Resident
Georgia Regents University

Foreword

As has been said by many, there is no greater privilege and no more challenging responsibility than to direct the care of those who are ill. More than knowledge, it requires competency, and more than competency it requires virtue, and more than virtue it requires both passion and compassion for another human being in distress. As an internal medicine residency program director for more than 25 years, it has been my joy to observe curious, empathetic, and disciplined students develop into wonderfully compassionate and consummate clinicians. They do this by focusing fully on their patients and their well being as men and women made in the Image of God, rather than data sets. Medicine is much more than making a diagnosis, prescribing a therapy, and offering a prognosis; it is a journey with another soul, sometimes for a shift, a day, a week, or decades.

Dr. Sayed's guidebook offers a convenient roadmap for the beginning of this journey. It is patient, rather than disease centered, and should be used as a starting point for the practice based learning and patient care competencies as well as virtues associated with hospital care and discharge planning. It is compact, convenient, and clear in its approach to the most common symptoms and problems of patients in modern hospitals.

Two things should be recognized by the reader, however: 1) Most hospitalized patients have more than one problem. They have multiple co-morbidities that include multiple diseases, social-economic, and especially psychological and even spiritual complexities that defy simple analysis and interact to thwart simplistic interventions. 2)

Situations in which patients find themselves are always dynamic and changing, with a past which may be hidden (especially childhood trauma and abuse), a presence which needs systemic understanding, and a future which depends on timeliness and follow through of plans made. This reference is a fine start for the genesis of an outstanding clinician. Savvy students will initiate a lifetime habit of frequent and lengthy visits to both the bedside and the enlarging greater body of literature. In each location they will ponder deeply both the causes and the effects of what is happening to their patients. Then, with experience, time, and devotion, they will be able also to taste and give to others the fruits of their practice.

David R. Haburchak, M.D. FACP
Professor of Medicine
Georgia Regents University

Life is short and art long, Opportunity fleeting,
Experience perilous and decision difficult.
Hippocrates

1. Antibiotics (abx)

The best abx choice is to send a good culture specimen for sensitivity & choose the PO form (or the IV form at first & then switch to PO as indicated) w/ consideration of the side effect, expense, frequency, & comorbidity. You can follow up the infx resolution & the abx effectiveness by monitoring the fever, Sx, ESR/CPR, WBC & clinical improvement. <u>Know what you are treating</u>.

Common used abx

- **Vancomycin**: 1st line G + broad coverage, good for MRSA. IV form for broad coverage especially for sepsis or confirmed gram+ infx like strep & staph including MRSA. PO form is only for c diff infx as it does NOT absorb in GI track. Follow up blood troughs (usually after the 3rd dose) & adjust dose accordingly (therapeutic 15-20mcg/ml). Dosing is mostly BID for normal kidney but should be changed to either daily or q48hrs for AKI or CKD stage ≥ III (pharmacy can help dosing). On dialysis, give the dose after the session & get trough before it as 30% will be dialyzed out. Common empiric therapy w/ Zosyn.
- **Clindamycin:** gram + & anaerobic, PO for anaerobic infx mainly below the diaphragm like abscess, mild cellulitis out pt, aspiration PNA. Effective against community MRSA (althoughdoxycline & bactrim is better). Weak against group B strep & ↑risk of c. diff.
- **Daptomycin**: IV, Gram positive. Usually is NOT the 1st choice & is used when Vanc fails as it has great MRSA coverage. Do NOT use for respiratory infx (due to pulmonary surfactant inhibition effect on Daptomycin, but it is good for osteomyelitis & skin infx). Is NOT aminoglycoside.
- **Zosyn (Pipercellin/Tazobactam):** IV form, 1st line broad-spectrum coverage (Gram+, - & anerobic), for moderate & severe infx like nosocomial PNA,

abdomen infx (diverticulitis, abscess & peritonitis), skin infx. Does NOT cover MRSA. Can be used w/ Amikacin (aminoglycoside) to cover nosocomial pseudomonas. Common combination w/ Vanc as empiric Tx. **Same group:** Unasyn (Ampicillin/Sulbactam), which is good against G- in general (Unlike Zosyn; it does NOT cover Pseudomonase). Augmentin (Amoxicillin/Clavulanate) is PO & common for out-pt mild-moderate infx like bacterial pharyngitis & sinusitis, animal bites, mild cellulitis (including diabetic foot), lower respiratory infx, & pyelonephritis.

- **Rocephin (Ceftriaxone):** IV cephalosporin, 3rd G, broad coverage (G+ & -), weak against Pseudomonas & anaerobic (do NOT use). Does NOT cover enteroccus (All cephalosporins do NOT cover it) or MRSA. Used for meningitis (especially caused by S. Pneumonia or meningococcal), gonococcalinfx, & prophylactic after sexual assault, UTI, skin infx, pelvic inflammatory disease, bone infx, & CAP (in combination w/ azithromycin). **Same Group: Ceftaroline:** 5th G cephalosporin & covers all MRSA; even Vanc resistant. **Cefdinir & Cefixime:** PO 3rd G cephalosporins (good for out pt therapy)

- **Azithromycin (z pack):** common out pt PO abx for atypical PNA, bronchitis, & GPC. 5 tablets 250mg each in 4 days. 2tab 1st day & then once qdaily. Yellow greenish phlegm does NOT automatically mean z pack.

- **Keflex:** 1^{st}G cephalosporin, PO for G +. Treats bone infx, UTI, otitis media, Upper RTI, strep pharyngitis. Mainly for skin flora & surgery likes them for prophylaxis. Great for cellulitis strep infx (good for MSSA). **Same group: Ancef & Duricef**

- **Linozolid:** PO or IV, Gram + including MRSA & Enterococcus. No Gram- coverage. Usually is a

13

2nd line after Vanc, especially for vanc resistance enterococcus. **Treat:** CAP, HCAP & skin infx. Does NOT treat bacteremia (NOT bactericidal).

- **Ciprofloxacin:** great for G- & pseudomonas (NOT good for G+). Used also for gastroparesis (from long lasting diabetes, manifests as early satiety & N/V) to ↑ GI motility. Prolongs QT interval. Use for: UTI, GI infx, CAP. Usually orally but available IV. Same group: Moxifloxacin & Levofloxacine (respiratory quinolones), which are preferred for CAP (good for G+ compared to Ciprofloxacin).

- **Amphotericin B:** IV, for severe fungal infx, mainly for AIDS & neutropenia pt or any immunosuppressed pt w/ presumed fungal infx for empiric fungal coverage. Order fungal blood culture before initiation. Nephrotoxic, hydration before & while on the med. Monitor electrolytes & kidney function.

- **Fluconazole:** common anti-fungal po drug for either Tx of common fungal infx especially candida (like PO thrush, vaginal candidiasis is, & even more severe cases like cryptococcal meningitis in AIDS) or prophylactic for immunosuppressed pts like in BMT. High doses can treat fungemia. Diflucan 150mg one dose po is a common Tx for vaginal candidiasis w/ white cheesy discharge (Vaginal Miconazole is another option). **Nystatin** is good for Candida infx like vaginal w/ creamy discharge, PO w/ white painful lesions or thrush, & skin candida (or Tania) w/ white flaky red skin w/ itching (use w/ combination of steroid like **Betamethasone** for Symptomatic relief). **Clotrimazole** topical is also effective against candida & most of other topical fungal infx (including athlete foot). Same group: **Voriconazol** (good for mold like aspergillus as fluconazole does NOT cover mold) & **Itraconazol**: for presumed serious fungal infx (comes in PO form).

- **Acyclovir:** effective against shingles if administered in 72 hrs from the blistering to reduce pain & ↓ duration. Another indication: herpetic encephalitis & genital herpes. Hydrate well before & during Tx due to risk of AKI. Same group: **ganciclovir** (mainly for CMV infx)

- **Metronidazole (Flagyl):** anerobic, 1st choice for clostridium difficile infx, vaginal infx (vaginosis w/ thin fishy smelling discharge & trichomoniasis w/ greenish yellowish discharge), Colorecatal infx, Giardia & Amebia infx. Category B in pregnancy (A accepted, D life threatening). Avoid Alcohol & educate about metallic taste.
- **Amikacin:** Aminoglycoside IV covers G- mainly. Treat: UTI, meningitis (G- infx), HCAP including Pseudomonas respiratory infx. Have nephro, neuro, & ototoxicity side effects. **Same group: Gentamycin & Tobramycin** (the best for pseudomonas & G-)
- **Doripenem:** broad coverage (GPC, GNB, & anerobic) except MRSA. From carbapenem group. Good for pseudomonas (intubation associated PNA or VAP). Only IV & is NOT usually 1st line Tx. Usually switched to it from zosyn if it fails for possible resistance (great gram negative coverage). At the same group: **Meropenem** which↑ risk of seizure in pt w/ CNS problem & **Ertapenem**, which is NOT covering pseudomonas but still good broad coverage (used once daily IV).
- **Aztreonam (monobactam abx):** IV/IM broad coverage for G- including pseudomonas aeruginosa (NOT good for G+ or anerobic). It is a synthetic monocyclic beta-lactam antibiotic (a monobactam). It is usually NOT the first line & used when other agents fail covering G- infx (like for UTI). Good option for penicillin allergy (cross reactivity is very low)
- **Bactrim:** Sulfa drug, usually PO. Very common use: PCP infx (& prophylactically) in immunosuppressed pts, UTI (lower for 3 days & upper use IV or PO for longer time, around 14days), skin (& soft tissue infx), CA-MRSA, &

15

COPD exacerbation. Caution w/ sulfa allergy & in pregnancy (category C).

Special considerations:

- **Good culture specimens**
    - ○ **Sputum:** Squamous epithelial cells line the mouth. If> 10 of these cells are present in the specimen then it is may be sputum w/ saliva but if<10 per hpf & >25 PMNs in the specimen, it is more likely to be from the lungs. Consider bronchoscopy by pulm for good sputum samples, if needed.
    - ○ **Urine:** mid-stream clean catch (foley cath is NOT a good sample as it is may be colonized w/ bacteria).
    - ○ **Abscess:** the wall of the cavity & NOT the pus (which is WBC & debris & may NOT have bacteria growing).
    - ○ **Osteomyelitis:** Cx curettage from the ulcer base following superficial debridement of necrotic tissue. Organisms cultured from superficial swabs are NOT reliable for predicting the pathogens responsible for deeper infx. Bone biopsy & Cx is important before Abx (especially in chronic osteo)

> **Attention:** Findings that indicate abx are failing (need to switch abx for possible resistance) → persistent fever after 48-72 hrs, clinical deterioration, worsening erythema (like for cellulitis if it's pen marked)

- **MRSA abx:** Vancomycin, Daptomycin, Ceftaroline & Linezolid (for hospital acquired MRSA) & Doxcycyline, Bactrim, Rifampin & Clinamycin (for community acquired MRSA).

16

Pseudomonas abx: Zosyn, cipro/Levofloxacin, Cefepime, Ceftazidime, Mero/Imi/Doripenem (Ertapenem is NOT good for Pseudomonas), Topramycin/Gyntamycin/Amikacine, Aztreonam, Fasfamycin, & Colistin

- **Same bioavailability if they are given IV or PO:** Azithromycin, Levofloxacin, Ciprofloxacin, doxycycline, clindamycin, linezolid, & fluconazole.
- **You can choose either IV or PO abx** depending on the specific infx you are treating. Endocarditis may need IV abx for 6 weeks (PICC line will be useful) but treating something like PNA or UTI→ it's ok to start IV & switch to PO or even begin w/ PO. PO intolerance makes IV rout a good option. For bacteremia start IV & check for one negative blood Cx. After 2-3 days switch to PO if negative.
- **Antimicrobial stewardship program** (program for wise abx use) De-escalation of therapy, IV to PO conversions, Dose optimization, Guidelines & clinical pathways, Education (Colonization vs. infx). Implementation of an antimicrobial stewardship program helps: Improve pt outcomes, Improve pt safety, Reduces resistance, & Reduces cost

2. Clostridium difficile infection (CDI)

C. difficile infx is a major cause of in pt gastrointestinal illness. C. difficile is a gram-positive, spore-forming, normal flora of the GI tract mostly spread by the fecal-PO route. Soap & water is the best for prophylaxis (alcohol foam does NOT eliminate spores).

Risk factors
Recent abx use is the main culprit, especially clindamycin, cephalosporins, & fluoroquinolones. Though, any abx can predispose to *C. difficile* overgrowth, including Vanc & metronidazole. Nursing home pts, elderly, immunosuppressed, & pts w/ altered GI anatomy (e.g., ileostomy, colostomy) are at ↑ risk.

Clinical features
Typical presentation is profuse watery diarrhea, lower abdominal pain/tenderness, & often extremely foul-smelling stool (nurses usually suspect that first).

Laboratory tests
The most accurate test is stool *C. difficile* antigen PCR. The disadvantage is that it takes around 24-48 hrs to return from the lab. Get CBC & CMP to assess severity.

Classification
Used to decide on Tx options, including possible ICU care.
- **Mild:** Diarrhea is the sole Sx.
- **Moderate:** Diarrhea plus additional signs & Sx NOT meeting criteria for severe or complicated CDI.
- **Severe:** Hypoalbuminemia (albumin <3), a WBC count >15 k, & abdominal tenderness.
  Complicated CDI pts who need to be considered for ICU: HoTN w/ or w/o vasopressors, fever > 38. 5°C, ileus, abdominal

distension, mental status changes, WBC count >35, 000or <2, 000, serum lactate level >2. 2 mmol/L, & any signs of end-organ failure.

Tx

Can be initiated before laboratory confirmation for pts w/ a ↑ pre-test suspicion. The offending abx should be stopped. If abx must be continued, treat w/ abx less known for causing CDI, such as aminoglycosides, macrolides, Vanc, or tetracycline.

- **For mild-to-moderate CDI**: PO metronidazole 500mg TID x10 days should be used. If the pt fails to respond to metronidazole therapy, a change in therapy to PO Vanc should be considered.
- **Severe or complicated disease:**
  w/o ileus → PO Vanc is administered (in addition to IV metronidazole)
  w/ ileus →Vanc delivered PO & per rectum plus IV metronidazole is to be given. Additionally, supportive care w/ fluid resuscitation, electrolyte replacement, & DVT prophylaxis should be continued. A CT abdomen & pelvis is recommended in pts w/ complicated CDI, as is a surgical consult due to possible need for subtotal colectomy & ileostomy, which is associated w/ ↓ mortality.
- **Recurrent disease:** The **first recurrence** of CDI should be treated w/ the same regimen used for the initial episode. However, if infx is severe, PO Vanc should be used. The **second recurrence** should be treated w/ Vanc PO. For a **third recurrence** after a pulsed Vanc regimen, fecal microbiota transplant (FMT) should be considered.

Special considerations
- **Fidaxomicin** was approved for mild-to-moderate CDI & was non-inferior to Vanc in phase III trials & **Fecal microbiol transplant (FMT)** has shown promising results in trials for recurrent CDI as mentioned above.

19

> **Attention**: Probiotics are NOT recommended according to current guidelines, especially in immunosuppressed pts, where there are a few case reports of bacteremia resulting from their use.

- **PO Vanc is expensive** but PO metronidazole is cheap.
- **Do NOT test C. diff in pts w/o diarrhea** (unless you have another reason like leukocytosis w/o known source). Monitor response to Tx by decreasing bowel movement numbers per day. Recovery is monitored clinically (usually no need to test negative C. diff as it can be positive after the Tx for months w/o the need to repeat abx & it is NOT a sign of Tx failure).
- **Start counting 14 days of anti C diff abx (like Flagyl or Vanc) from the time you stop the offending agent** (like Clindamycin). Do NOT undertreat in order to avoid recurrence.

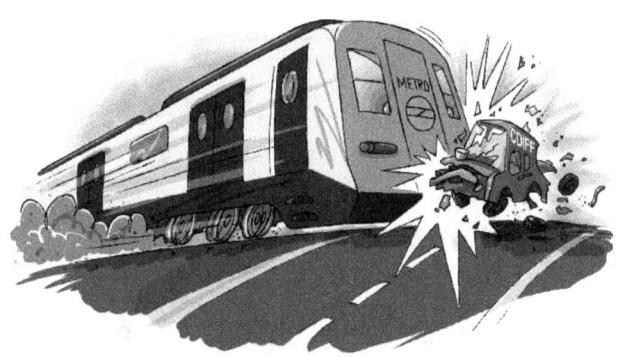

METROnidazole is effective against C diff infx.

3. Methicillin-Resistant Staphylococcus Aureus (MRSA)

Thisis a major cause of morbidity & mortality in hospitals. It can cause PNA, bacteremia & skin & skin structure infx (SSSIs). Tx has become challenging because of resistance & limited availability of antimicrobial agents. Moreover, there has been an emergence of community-acquired strains (CA-MRSA), which sometimes have a higher virulence than hospital-acquired ones.

Community-acquired MRSA

Clindamycin, trimethoprim-sulfamethoxazole (TMP-SMX) & tetracyclines (doxycycline) are recommended as first line agents for CA-MRSA, but should NOT be used for hospital-acquired strains due to ↑ resistance. Out of the 3 agents mentioned above, only clindamycin has good activity against both MRSA & beta-hemolytic Streptococci. Usually, in skin infx thought to be due to MRSA, empiric coverage for both MRSA & Streptococci is needed. However, using clindamycin as a sole agent can lead to resistance. Hence, TMP-SMX or doxycycline in combination w/ a beta-lactam agent, such as ampicillin or amoxicillin, is preferred.

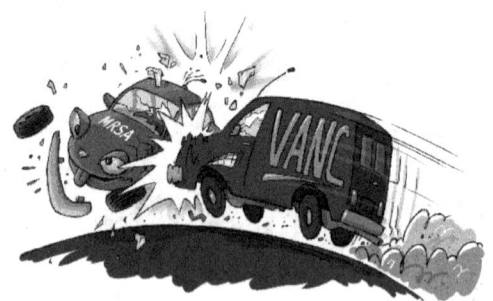

*VANcomycin is the 1ˢᵗ empiric IV Tx of choice for **MRSA**; especially for in pt.*

> **Attention**: Clindamycin is associated w/ a relatively higher risk for *c diff infx.*

Hospital-acquired MRSA: Nursing homes, dialysis centers, or any long-term healthcare facility. Has been treated w/ IV **Vanc** for several years. It is cheap, effective, & has years of experience behind its use as a first line agent. However, in recent years, there have been reports of ↑ resistance & rising minimum inhibitory concentrations (MICs).

There are several reports of emergence of VRSA (Vanc resistant *S. aureus*), VISA (Vanc intermediate *S. aureus*), & HVRSA (heterogeneous Vanc resistant *S. aureus*). However, as of now, it is still used as a first line agent for MRSA.
Vanc is a bactericidal agent & acts by inhibiting cell wall synthesis. It is used only in IV formulation (unless specifically treating *C. difficile* infx), & requires dose adjustment in renal insufficiency. Nephrotoxicity & red man syndrome are among the most common adverse effects associated w/ it, & require stopping the drug. Trough (blood level) should be checked regularly to assure therapeutic levels (make sure it is a true trough by checking it just before the next dose or before HD).

Linezolid is another agent that can be used in both PO & IV formulations. It has good lung penetration & is recommended for MRSA PNA NOT responding well to Vanc & in pts being discharged back to a nursing home on PO meds.

Daptomycin is among the newer agents approved for Tx of MRSA. It is used for MRSA bacteremia, but is NOT recommended for use in MRSA PNA as it is inactivated by pulm surfactant. Additionally, it can be used for complicated skin infx & infective endocarditis. Adverse effects include myopathy (monitor CPK), peripheral neuropathy, & eosinophilic PNA.

Ceftaroline (Cephalosporins) is good for MRSA & is approved for PNA & cellulitis infx (NOT the 1st line though)

4. Volume Overload

A diagnosis of overloaded volume status can be elicited by a good h & p. It can be attributed to CHF (systolic mostly but also diastolic w/ preserved EF), cirrhosis, or nephropathy in most cases. In the in pt setting, volume overload is often iatrogenic caused simply by too much IV fluid or over-resuscitated truly hypovolemic pts (failure to adjust fluid infusion rate from replacement fluid deficit to maintenance rate). Often it is hard to assess volume status accurately.

History:
- **Ask about compliance w/ fluid restriction (1-1. 5 Liter) & ↓ Na$^+$ diet,** especially for CHF pts. Any Na rich food & processed foods, salty foods may NOT necessarily taste salty to the pt. This is especially common during or around the holidays (eating at restaurants, canned foods, fried foods, etc).
- **Ask about meds compliance:** Have they skipped any doses of meds recently? Ask this question particularly to pts on diuretics who have complained about ↑ urinary frequency as a side effect. Also ask if they have been adjusting their Lasix or diuretic dose depending on their daily weight (Do they have scale at home)?
- **Have they taken or been prescribed any new meds recently?** One common culprit is NSAIDs (associated w/ worsening heart failure/HTN & of course worsening CKD).
- **Ask about missing dialysis** it is a common cause for volume overload & SOB/pulm edema hospital admissions. Always ask about recent weight change.

Exam & tests:
- Pts w/ volume status issues should be examined multiple times per day to assess the rate of

diuresis or IV fluid infusion in case of hypo or hypervolemia (stop when pt is euvolemic).

- **Vitals:** especially BP (HoTN indicates poor LV function while elevated BP maybe the reason for diastolic or systolic CHF exacerbation).
- **Inspection:** ↑ daily weight, pitting edema which must be assessed over a bony surface such as the shins or metatarsals, pronounced neck veins & elevated JVP (↑ Sen. & Spec.) & be on the alert for IV fluids hanging in the pt's room that are flowing continuously when in fact these fluids should have been held. Dependent edema is commonly seen in bedridden or supine pts in flank regions.
- **Auscultation:** Crackles & rales, shifting dullness from ascites, high liver span assessed via percussion, S3 heart sound due to turbulent blood flow from high volume (gallop)
- **CXR:** to establish a baseline w/ serial x-rays to assess improvement in the case of pulm edema (CXR changes occur quickly in comparison to PNA infiltrations). Remember to look at the CXR yourself to assess for Kerley B lines, hilar haze, cephalization of pulm vasculature, thickening of pleural fissures, peribronchial cuffing, diffuse opacification (AKA complete white out), & pleural effusion.
- **TTE:** should be considered up front to evaluate & compare ejection fraction or at least establish a baseline.
- **RUQ ultrasound:** to evaluate for hepatomegaly & congestion.
- **Labs:** Serum Cr (elevated Cr usually indicates renal involvement which could be either AKI or ESRD w/ missed HD) & BNP (elevated BNP indicates volume overload).

Management:

For all pts: stop IV fluids & consider mnemonic LMNOP (Lasix, Morphine, nitrates, O_2, posture), which is basically Tx for pulm edema (pt is sick & needs emergent Tx). Also, recommend a ↓Na diet, fluid restriction, record daily ins & outs, encourage strict meds & HD compliance (if applicable).

For ESRD pts who have missed HD, arrange for dialysis, consult nephrology, & educate regarding compliance.

For cirrhosis pts w/ ascites, assess the need for therapeutic paracentesis & replace albumin (25 ml of albumin for every 2 liters of ascitic fluid removed).

Special considerations:

- **Pulmonary edema or congestion can occur w/o signs of peripheral edema** (lower extremities swelling, JVD, & hepatojugular reflex), especially if the etiology is HTN urgency/emergency w/ CHF & vice versa, peripheral edema can occur w/o pulm edema. The cornerstone of Tx is diuresis, especially for peripheral edema as these pts may sometimes have 10-20 liters of extra volume that needs to be eliminated.

> **Attention:** Pts w/ pulm edema from uncontrolled HTN w/o peripheral edema can be euvolumic (or even volume depleted from chronic diuresis) & diuresis should be brief along w/ controlling BP.

- **The physical examination** of pts who are volume depleted is often less telling than that of their overloaded counterparts.
- **Diuresis should be targeted** to achieve daily negative fluid balance. Net negative of 0.5-1L is usually safe, & might need to be more when

patient is symptomatic. Always check BMP (for K & Cr), Mg, & phosphate, & correct electrolyte abnormality as needed (Q 12 hrs). It is highly recommended to supplement K^+ & Mg^{2+} orally in the case of a high diuresis target, even if they are normal (prophylactically).

- **Usually loop diuresis w/ Lasix or Bumex either orally or IV** (PO meds do NOT absorb effectively due to intestinal edema in volume overload pts) is adequate. If the response is suboptimal, you can add thiazide diuretics like metolazone (once a day 30 minutes before the loop diuretic dose) for a synergetic effect.

- **Monitor serum Cr closely** as risk of AKI is a common consequence of overdiuresis. ↓diuretic dose (or even stop it) in case of Cr elevation (↓ urine output is another indicator for volume depletion). ↓central venous pressure (CVP) in ICU pts w/ a central line (normal CVP is 8-12) is a good sign of volume depletion (low CVP is almost always a sign of low volume status & indicating need for IV fluid).

> **Attention:** measure CVP "by yourself" as it is an essential value and you need it to be accurate.

- **NOT all edema or ascites needs diuresis** such as in the case of cirrhosis or malnutrition. In these cases, low oncotic pressure intravascularly causes "leakage" of the fluid into the interstitial space (third space). Pt's intravascular volume might be low & diuretics may NOT help. Measure CVP (if central line is available in the ICU) & urine Na. You may need to give IV fluid in the case of persistent low BP, ↓ CVP, ↓ urine Na^+ & signs of poor end organ perfusion, such as AKI. Improving nutrition may ↓ the edema (albumin infusion is expensive & does NOT help due to the short half life).

5. Volume Depletion

Most cases of volume depletion can be attributed to an etiology of gastrointestinal losses, renal losses, skin losses, third space sequestration, or iatrogenic causes.

H & P:

- GI loss like diarrhea or vomiting? GI bleeding indicated by either BRBPR or black, tarry stool? ↓ PO fluid intake for any reason such as an elderly pt w/ AMS, NPO w/o IV fluid, or excessive sweating? Finally: consider pancreatitis, trauma such as crush injuries (Which could reveal pancreatic injury), recent surgery, or abdominal pain that could indicate peritonitis. All of these etiologies could contribute to third spacing.

- **Vitals→** tachycardia (first sign usually but maybe masked by AV node blocking agents) & HoTN. Tachypnea for any reason can ↑ insatiable water loss & cause volume depletion.

- Helpful equations to know:
  MAP=CO x TPR
  CO= HR x SV
  MAP= HR x SV x TPR
  HR= MAP/SV x TPR.

  (Mean artery pressure MAP, Cardiac output CO, Total peripheral resistance TPR, Heart rate HR, Stroke volume SV).

- **Inspection:** malaise, fatigue, thirst, muscle cramping, syncope, postural dizziness, abdominal & CP due to ischemia of the mesenteric or coronary vasculature, confusion, & altered mental status due to ↓ cerebral vascular perfusion. Assess skin turgor or lack thereof & delayed capillary refill. Tachypnea may be present due to acidosis. Muscular irritability (or cramps) & confusion may be present due to metabolic alkalosis. Muscle weakness & cramping may be observed due to hyperkalemia or hypokalemia. Seizures & coma may occur due to hyponatremia or hypernatremia. Flattened neck veins may be noted.

- **Auscultation→**Listen for groaning & moaning due to abdominal pain or CP as well as muscle cramping. Pts may tell you that they have been urinating more or even less frequently (due to AKI/ dehydration). Tachycardia & tachypnea may be present as mentioned above.
- **Labs: Check BMP** (elevated Cr usually indicates overdiuresis & intravascular volume depletion). Check **urine electrolytes** (urine Na & urine Cr along w/ BMP) & calculate **FeNa** (calculator **available online**) or **FeUrea** if pt is on diuresis (get urine Cr & urine Urea along w/ BMP). Calculate the **BUN to Cr ratio** (high in dehydration). Check **lactic acid** level to assess for lactic acidosis (usually q4-6hrs until resolution).

Management: IV hydration (mostly normal saline): start w/ few liters boluses (as needed) & then keep maintenance fluid (if can NOT tolerate PO).

Attention:
1. Dehydration is different than hypovolemia although they are treated mostly the same. Hypovolemia "low blood volume", which is NOT identical to dehydration "loss of water" because blood is NOT pure water.
2. FeNa (&even FeUrea) are very helpful to diagnose the etiology of **oliguria**. FeNa <1% → prerenal (Tx mostly w/ hydration) vs >1→renal/post-renal. FeNa is NOT very helpful in case of normal UOP.

---

6. Pain

Is often considered the fifth vital sign. It is one of the most common complaints of pts admitted in the hospital & often, incorrectly managed. It is a subjective sensation & hence, hard to reliably quantify.

Classification & Management: Pain can be measured by VAS scale (0-10, 10 being the worst). Mild (1-3) usually needs Tylenol/NSAIDs, moderate (4-7) usually needs oral opioids (Percocet or lortab)/tramadol (w/ or w/o Tylenol/ NSAIDs) & severe (8-10) usually needs IV opioids. As pain is very subjective & pain tolerance is different; above formulas can be adjusted accordingly. Another classification is the chronicity of the pain (acute or chronic)

   A. **Acute pain** (Postoperative pain, inflammation, trauma, burns, & sickle cell crisis): Usually lasts for a few days. Try to eliminate the source before starting the pt on a pain meds regimen. 1st line agents are non-narcotic analgesics such as acetaminophen & non-steroidal anti-inflammatory drugs (NSAIDs). They are most effective for mild to moderate pain, pain related to inflammation, musculoskeletal pain, & HAs. All NSAIDs inhibit cyclooxygenase (COX), usually both 1 & 2. The COX-1 enzyme is also expressed in the epithelium of the GI tract & hence, non-selective COX inhibitors can cause GI toxicity (ulcers & gastritis; take after food). There are non-selective COX-2 inhibitors, such as Celecoxib, but they are rarely used due to the ↑ risk of adverse cardiovascular events. Chronic use of COX-2 inhibitors has been reported to ↑ death from myocardial infarction. Some have IV formulations. Two of these IV formulations include IV ketorolac & IV acetaminophen, which are effective in avoiding or reducing the requirement of opioids.

Adverse effects: GI irritation, interstitial nephritis, NSAIDs nephropathy (including AKI due to inhibition of renal prostaglandins), & HTN w/ chronic use (Naproxen is maybe the safest). **Use w/ caution:** acetaminophen in hepatic impairment (use lower doses, usually <2 g/day). **Contraindications of NSAIDs usage:** renal insufficiency, CHF (still used/ Naproxin is preferred), GI bleed (or recent hx w/ caution), post-operative state (most of them, except Tylenol have an anti-platelet effect & also delay wound healing).

B. **Chronic pain (Cancer, terminal illness, neuropathic pain, & certain pain syndromes such as fibromyalgia):** Pts in continuous pain require round-the-clock analgesia. Usually long-acting opioids are give n at a basal dose w/ short-acting ones given as needed (PRN) at 10-20% of the basal dose. If frequent PRN doses are used, they should be added up & a new basal dose is calculated.

Opioids: Inadequate dosing w/ opioids is one of the most common errors made by physicians & leads to unnecessary suffering. Also, there is reluctance to use opioids due to unsubstantiated fear of addiction when evidence points out the fact that use of opioids for a genuine cause of pain rarely fosters addiction. Also, the physician should develop an opioid management plan or 'pain contract' w/ pts (mostly in out pt setting). This typically includes stipulations that pain meds will NOT be sought elsewhere, pt will abstain from illicit drugs, will keep clinic appointments as scheduled, & will obtain random urine drug screens.

A copy of this signed document is given to the pt & reviewed periodically during follow-up visits. Usually short-acting opioids such as morphine, Percocet (oxycodone/acetaminophen), loratab (hydrocodone/acetaminophen) are preferred in acute pain. Long-acting formulations such as MS Contin, Oxycontin controlled release, methadone, fentanyl patches (NOT preferred as 1st line) are reserved for chronic pain.

Adjuvant pain therapy:

- **Anticonvulsants** (gabapentin, pregabalin & valproate) & anti-depressants (amitriptyline, desipramine, duloxetine & venlafaxine) are considered 1st line drugs in neuropathic pain. Tricyclic anti-depressants are usually avoided because of adverse effects, mostly their anticholinergic effects. Gabapentin is usually started 1st (start w/ small dose & titrate up).

- **Muscle relaxant** like flexeril, Suboxone & baclofen (avoid driving car while on them) are preferred to treat muscle spasms in the neck, Back & extremities. Muscle pain usually is severe, non- radiating & associated usually w/ hrs to days hx of heavy lifting or excessive exercise. NSAIDs also can be used along w/ topical pain creams (like Diclofenac topical, Lidocaine patch, & Capsaicin cream) & hot massage.

- Consider **Physical therapy PT & exercise programs** (especially aquatic therapy for elderly w/ balance issues) for chronic pain like Fibromyalgia & chronic pain syndrome, as it can be very effective w/ Cognitive therapy. PT can also strengthen the muscles around the joints & ↓ osteoarthritis pain (especially knees & back pain)

Special consideration:

- **Addiction:** Opioid drug abuse is a common problem & steps must be taken by every health care professional to curb it. Pain meds should be prescribed by one health care practitioner & the pt must be bound by a "pain contract".

32

Judicious use of opioids & making every effort to wean pts off them would go a long way in dealing w/ this issue (narcotics prescribed for any reason ↑ mortality comparing to normal population).

> **Attention:** scheduled pain meds are preferred over "PRN" in order to ↓ addiction & ↑ efficacy. Add "PRN" at the top of scheduled meds in specific cases. Educate pt that pain may not go to zero &<3 is maybe acceptable in chronic pain.

- **Pt-controlled analgesia PCA:** a system through which the pt self-administers predetermined doses of opioids. Morphine & dilaudid are two commonly used drugs for PCA, & is usually used in pts requiring large doses of opioids, such as those w/ chronic pain syndromes, like sickle cell disease. PCA can administer a basal dose (at a continuous hourly rate) & bolus doses (which is administered by the pt) w/ a lockout interval (which can be adjusted, usually from 7-20 minutes). Advantages of a PCA include greater pain relief, pt satisfaction, & fewer complications.
- **Always prevent ileus/constipation** by starting bowel regimen (colace, Miralax, ± stimulants like Senna). Relistor (Methylnaltrexone) is an opioid reversal agent in the GI system (expensive; try to avoid the need for it). Urinary retention is an opioid side effect like constipation but maybe less common (NOT preventable).
- **Respiratory suppression** is an opioid side effect & it happen due to hypoventilation (↓ respiratory rate); so SOB & O_2 desaturation should be assessed in pts on opioids. Respiratory rate of 30-40 may NOT indicate an

opioid overdose. In general: avoid meds can ↓ mental status (like benzos or opioids) in pts who has respiratory distress or O_2 desaturation (for any reason) to avoid the need for intubation. Narcan is the opioid antidote (fast response).

- **Oxycodone** (w/o the Tylenol) has a high street value & drug abusers can use it by sniffing & IV for euphoria effects
- **Conversion of opioids** derivatives from type to another & from route to another (PO →IV or IV →PO) is **available online**. Chronic opioid users may need more than the calculated IV dose when converting from PO due to tolerance. Starting opioid doses should be lower for elderly.
- **Fentanyl** is NOT preferred for narcotic Naïve pts. **Methadon** has a lot of formulas (like tablets, oral solution, IV,etc) & it is common in hospice care.
- **Opioids rotation:** means changing the opioid type over time to ↓ side effect with prolonged use.

7. Diabetes mellitus (DM)

Diabetes Mellitus (DM) is a common metabolic disturbance seen in U. S adults & occurs due to a defect in insulin secretion, action, or both. Around 11% of the U. S population >20 years old is affected. Around 90% of those cases belong to the type II category.

Classification: The majority of cases can be classified into one of two categories: type I (<10%) & type II (>90%). Other specific types of DM exist related to certain genetic defects, drugs, endocrinopathies, & other syndromes. Also, DM related to pregnancy is known as gestational diabetes mellitus (resolved after delivery, recurrent in subsequent gestations, & can become overt DM).

Diagnosis: suggested by any of the following criteria:
1. Plasma glucose > 126 mg/dl after an overnight fast (should be confirmed w/ a repeat test). Fasting glucose level between 100-125 mg/dl indicates Impaired Fasting Glucose (IFG).
2. Random glucose level > 200 mg/dl plus Sx of diabetes mellitus (polyuria, polydipsia, fatigue, weight loss). Values of 140-199 mg/dl indicate Impaired Glucose Tolerance (IGT).
3. PO glucose tolerance test, which shows a glucose level > 200 mg/dl 2 hrs after administration of a 75 gm glucose load.
4. HgbA1c>6. 5% (needs to be confirmed w/ any of the above).

Management: Glycemic control & management of other atherosclerosis risk factors like HTN (JNC-8 guidelines, target has changed to BP <140/90), HLD (LDL goal is <100 mg/dl), smoking, & monitor for diabetic end organ damage such as retinopathy & glomerulopathy (by early referral to ophthalmology, w/ in 10 years for type I & on the time of diagnoses for type II, & referral to nephrology in CKD stage III). Fasting CBG should be between 70 to 130 mg/dl & postprandial CBG should be targeted to <180 mg/dl w/ Hgb A1c < 7%. For in pt (especially critically ill pts) target CBG should NOT be strictly controlled → okay <180 to avoid hypoglycemia. Consider more strict A1c control (<5.5%) in CF & pregnant pts. **DM Type I:** Type I requires lifelong insulin replacement. The sooner DM II is diagnosed, the more insulin secreting beta cells will be saved from destruction & the easier DM will be managed.

Type of insulin	Onset of action (hrs)	Peak effect (hrs)	Effect duration (hrs)
Rapid acting			
Lispro/Aspart/Glulisi-ne	<15min	≈1	3-5
Regular (draw 1st in syringe if mixed w/ NPH)	≈1	2-4	6-8
Intermediate acting			
NPH (only one cloudy, rest clear)	≈1.5	6-8	12-16
Long acting			
Glargine	1-2	0	Up to 24
Levemir/Detemir	1-2	0	Up to 24

Usually, in an average pt, total daily dose (TDD) of insulin is calculated by the following formula: 0.2-0.8 units/kg per day (0. 2 units/kg is usually started in a newly diagnosed/insulin naive pt). About 50% of the dose is usually basal insulin (intermediate or long-acting insulin, either NPH twice daily or detemir/glargine once daily), & the rest can be divided to three times/day before meals (or even twice depending on the compliance).

Two of the most commonly used regimens are:
1. **NPH & regular (2-3 injections/day):** Calculate Total Daily Dose TDD as per 0.4-0.8 units/kg. Divide it ½ & ½ OR $2/3^{rd}$ & $1/3^{rd}$ in morning & evening, depending on the biggest meal in the day. Divide the morning dose administered w/ breakfast into $2/3^{rd}$ NPH & $1/3^{rd}$ regular.

   Divide the evening dose into ½ NPH (to be administered at bedtime) & ½ regular (to be administered w/ evening meal). Then, calculate the correction factor by the following formula: 1700 divided by the TDD. This means that 1 unit of insulin will bring down the glucose by approximately x mg (x-correction factor, try to make the numbers easy to calculate like 50, 60, etc.). **Correction factor calculation is time consuming & can be avoided safely most of the time.**

   This regimen is also the cheapest available on the market. It is a good regimen for non-insured, newly diagnosed DM, & non-compliant pts as it needs fewer sticks.
   NPH & regular insulin can be prescribed also as a pre-mixed combination of 70% NPH/30% regular regimen (commonly known as 70/30) & it can be given twice daily (before breakfast & lunch or lunch & dinner, depends on the two largest meals)

2. **Glargine & aspart/lispro/regular (four times a day regimen):** Usually 50% of TDD is administered as long-acting glargine at night, & the remaining dose is divided into 3 times a day as rapid acting insulin given w/ meals.

   Supplemental sliding scale SSS can be added to the scheduled doses for better DM control (increase the scheduled insulin dose according to the previous day requirement from the SSS).

CBGs should be monitored both as an in pt & as an out pt at least 3-4 times/day (2 times is acceptable for out pt). Monitoring should include fasting CBG pre-breakfast & random post-prandial checks (writing them in a log can help in adjusting insulin doses).

Type II DM: Initial therapy is w/ PO agents. **Metformin** is commonly used as it has an added benefit of reducing obesity (↓ mortality as well). Also, it does NOT cause hypoglycemia (adverse reactions: N/V, & diarrhea). However, it should be used w/ caution in pts w/ renal disease (avoid in CKDIII or more as it could cause lactic acidosis). Sulfonylureas (SFU) such as glipizide, glyburide, & glimepiride are also used commonly.

Other non-SFU analogues such as nateglinide & repaglinide are rarely used. Other options include alpha-glucosidase inhibitor acarbose, thiazolidinediones such as rosiglitazone or pioglitazone (can cause fluid retention & should thus be used w/ caution in cardiac or renal disease), dipeptidyl peptidase-4 inhibitors sitagliptin & saxagliptin, bile acid sequestrant colesevelam, & glucagon-like peptide agonists such as exenatide. Eventually, type II DM pts end up needing insulin, which should be started as discussed above.

Diabetic ketoacidosis:
DKA occurs in up to 5% of pts w/ type I DM & can rarely occur in type II DM as well. It is often precipitated due to interruption of insulin dose when the pt feels sick. Precipitating factors could be a UTI, PNA, sepsis, MI, or trauma.
Usually include polyuria, polydipsia, N/V, abdominal pain, & signs of dehydration. Labs will show an elevated anion gap metabolic acidosis, elevated CBGs (however DKA can also rarely occur w/ normal CBGs), & electrolyte abnormalities.

Management:
Should include **fluid replacement therapy & insulin.**
Fluid replacement therapy is extremely important &
should be started w/o delay. There is a fluid deficit of
several liters, which should be replaced w/ normal saline
boluses until vital signs stabilize & urine output is
established.

After initial boluses, free water deficit is replaced w/
maintenance fluids (either normal saline or 0. 45% saline
at 150–500 ml/hr for severe hypernatremia; always
remember to correct Na for CBG).
Insulin therapy is usually started w/ initial fluid
replacement. A bolus of regular insulin at 0.1 units/kg is
given as soon as possible. Then, an insulin drip at 0.1
units/kg/hr is started. CBG should be lowered gradually
at a rate of 50-75 mg/dl/hr (excess rapid correction>100
mg/dl/hr can lead to osmotic encephalopathy).

BMP & CBGs need to be monitored every 2 hrs.
Once CBG reaches 250 mg/dL, fluids should be
changed to dextrose (5%) in 0. 45% saline to prevent
dangerous hypoglycemia.

**Insulin drip is continued until anion gap closes & pt
has clinically improved.** Subcutaneous insulin is
usually started once pt starts eating. Always remember
to continue the insulin drip for an hr after administration
of subcutaneous insulin as it takes time to take effect.

Potassium: K deficit should always be anticipated, even
if initial BMP shows normal K, as insulin administration
can cause shift of K intracellularly. K should be routinely
added to IV fluids at a rate of 10-20 meq/hr except in pts
w/ hyperkalemia (>6 mmol/hr), renal failure, or oliguria.
Bicarbonate, phosphate, & Mg rarely need to be
replaced.

Bicarbonate: therapy in DKA is indicated only if pH <7. 1, shock/coma, plasma bicarbonate <5, acidosis-induced cardiorespiratory dysfunction, or severe hyperkalemia. When discharging pts w/ DKA, always remember to provide DM education to prevent further episodes.

Hyperosmolar non-ketotic syndrome (HONK):

Commonly seen in type II DM. It is very similar to DKA w/ some difference. HONK is typically more insidious in onset w/ dehydration (due to diuresis effect of the very high blood glucose) & some neurological deficits. No or mild ketoacidosis in HONK (PH >7.30 & HCO3 >15) compared to DKA (anion gab metabolic acidosis) due to the presence of insulin in the former (prevent lipolysis). **Tx:** same as DKA; especially **IV hydration.**

Hypoglycemia:

Common in the in pt setting & is often iatrogenic or caused by inadequate PO intake.

Management:

For conscious pts, orange juice, candy bars, fruits, & crackers can be given immediately (or Glucose tablets). IV dextrose should be used for pts w/ AMS. Initial bolus of 20 to 50 mL of 50% dextrose followed by an infusion D5W should be administered w/o delay. **Glucagon 1 mg IM/SC** can be administered for those who are unable to take PO or who do NOT have IV access (or pts w/ "bad veins" & hard to get IV access on).

Complications of diabetes:

Long-term complications are divided into microvascular & macrovascular. Microvascular include diabetic retinopathy (usually the 1st one to occur), nephropathy, & neuropathy. Coronary artery disease & peripheral vascular disease are some of the macrovascular complications.

> **Attention**: Tight CBG control (A1c <6.5-7%)→ reduce microvascular complications w/ minimal to no benefit for macrovascular complications (so pts w/ CVA, PAD or CAD may target A1c 7-8, especially w/ hx of hypoglycemia). Young pts → A1c <6.5-7%.

Routine screening: Pts w/ newly diagnosed type II DM should get an ophthalmology referral (yearly) to screen for diabetic retinopathy (possible laser Tx for non/proliferative retinopathy or "leaky vessels" to prevent blindness). For type I DM, it is usually recommended 5 years after diagnosis. Urine microalbumin (yearly), lipid panel, neurological exam & detailed foot exam should be done in yearly basis or more often (PRN).

Special considerations:

- **ACE inhibitors or ARBs are recommended** as 1st line for HTN w/ DM as they are known to prevent renal complications.
- **Standard insulin concentration is 100 units/mL (U-100).** Rarely, a highly concentrated form of insulin U-500 (500 units/mL) is used (when you need a very high dose of U-100 like 100s)
- **Diabetes mellitus in hospitalized pts:** Numerous studies have been done on glycemic control in hospitalized pts. The generally accepted target is 140 for floor pts & 180 for ICU pts (or critically ill pts). Avoidance of hypoglycemia should be a priority in both ICU & non-ICU pts.
- **In general: Insulin should be started for all DM type I & DM type II if oral meds failed** to control A1c (<6.5 - 7%). Consider starting insulin for DM type II if A1c is very high on the initial presentation (like >10%) due to the fact that oral

meds ↓ A1c around 1% per one med (usually you can NOT use more than 3 oral meds). Certain compliant pts can still control their A1c with diet, exercise & oral meds even if A1c is >10 on the presentation.

- **Supplemental insulin (less preferred term is sliding scale insulin):** is commonly used in addition to the scheduled dose for in pt to better control CBG. For optimal DM management, scheduled doses should be adjusted in a daily bases (at AM) according to the previous day supplemental insulin doses (if the pt expected to have the same calorie intake). So if pt is scheduled for 5 U aspart before dinner & he/she took 2 U after dinner on the supplemental scale → give 7 U aspart instead of 5 U the next evening.
- **Hypoglycemia:** usually when CBG <50-60.
  Sx: AMS (even coma) and/or sympathetic nervous system stimulation (palpitation, sweating, & anxiety).
  Etiology: diabetics w/ insulin over dosing, skipping meals, oral diabetes meds (especially in setting of AKI or CKD), sepsis, adrenal insufficiency, EtOH or exercise (w/o ↓ insulin dose).
  Management: check A1c, cortisol, TSH, UDS, possible infx, & C peptide (exogenous insulin?). Consider glucose tolerance test, review meds (especially new ones) & prediabetes (in DMII when insulin resistance ↑ →reactive hypoglycemia from ↑ insulin secretion after meals →Tx w/ metformin!). Tx w/ PO sugary fluid, IV dextrose (amp of D50% or drip D5/D10).

"THE SILENT KILLERS"

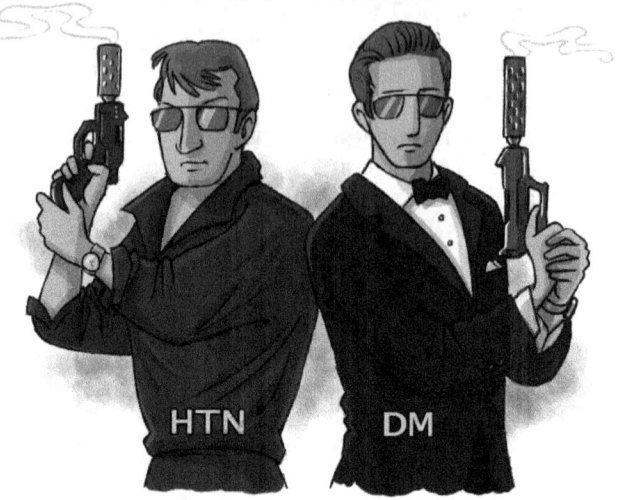

HTN & DM are the "silent killers" & may NOT cause symptoms. Treat & follow the numbers as appropriate.

8. Hypertension (HTN)

Primary HTN

Normal blood pressure		Systolic <120 mmHg & diastolic <80 mmHg
PreHTN		Systolic 120 to 139 mmHg or diastolic 80 to 89 mmHg
HTN	Stage 1	Systolic 140 to 159 mmHg or diastolic 90 to 99 mmHg.
	Stage 2	Systolic ≥160 or diastolic ≥100 mmHg

Management
Lifestyle modifications & drug therapy. Consider Na restriction, weight loss, dietary modification, exercise, & relaxation techniques. If lifestyle modifications have no effect over 3-6 months→initiate medical therapy (initiate meds if stage 2 directly)

Tx:
Consider comorbidities & drug adverse effects (DAE):
- **Thiazide diuretics** such as HCTZ or chlorthalidone (better than HCTZ) are very common. DAE: hyponatremia, ↑ Ca reabsorption (prevent osteoporosis) & ↑ uric acid reabsorption (worsen gout) in the kidney.
- **Diabetes:** use ACE-I/ARB (like lisinopril/losartan) as it protects the kidney & helps w/ proteinuria. DAE: AKI (in pts w/ CKD), ↑ K, cough, angioedema (tongue/throat/face swelling w/ SOB). Do NOT use if Cr>2. 5-3 or in renal artery stenosis. Monitor BMP (Cr & K) more frequent

when you first start ACEi/ARB (↑ in Cr <30% of baseline is expected due to the mechanism of action & meds should NOT be stopped just because of that). ACEi/ARB are contraindicated in pregnancy (do NOT prescribe if pt is trying to conceive, category D)

- **CAD:** use β blocker (metoprolol either short acting like titrate q12h or succinate q24h, atenolol, Coreg)
- **CHF:** use β blocker, ACE-I or ARB (if ACE-I is NOT tolerated, use ARB)
- **Migraine:** β blocker or CCB (it has prophylactic effects)
- **Hyperthyroidism:** β blocker (Propranolol)
- **Osteoporosis:** thiazide (because it reabsorbsCa) & avoid thiazide in gout (reabsorbs uric acid)
- **Pregnancy:** alpha methyldopa, labetalol, CCB, Clonidine (rebound HTN is common in case of sudden stoppage), thiazide diuretics & hydralazine (used IV for preeclampsia)
- **BPH:** alpha blocker (Prazosin or flomax)

If BP is NOT controlled w/ one drug, add a second drug: β blocker, ACE-I/ARB, CCB, sprinolactone, thiazide
If BP is still NOT controlled w/ the second drug, add a third drug (include diuretics if NOT already) & investigate for secondary HTN causes (preferably after 24 hrs continues BP monitor to confirm elevated BP).

Secondary HTN
Investigate for secondary HTN if you see the following: Young (<30) or old (>60) pt, refractory HTN (failure to control w/ 3 meds including diuretics), Bruit (renal artery stenosis), Episodic HTN (pheochromocytoma), Buffalo hump, truncal obesity, striae (Cushing's), Hypokalemia (Conn's), UE pressure>LE pressure (coarctation of the aorta), & Hirsutism (congenital adrenal hyperplasia)

Special considerations:
- **Start w/ two anti HTN meds** for pts w/ Stage 2 HTN & adjust doses in following visits (usually one med is NOT enough).
- **Check BP multiple times** (do NOT diagnose HTN from single reading), no caffeine, empty bladder, no tobacco or EtOH, relaxed, sitting down & try different devices if error suspected (or manually).
- **Every effort should be done to put pts on β blocker & ACE-I/ARB** due to the great mortality benefits they offer to diabetic & CHF pts. Escalate the doses as tolerated & check the heart rate for the β blocker (do NOT escalate if HR around 60) & the serum Cr for ACE-I.
- **Elderly Pts** especially w/ long-term DM & ESRD (stiff arteries due to calcification) experience hypotensive Sx on normal systolic BP readings like 110s-120s. De-escalate BP meds to achieve "new normal BP" in the range of 140s-150s.
- **HTN Emergency:** BP >210s/120s w/ end organ damage (like AMS, AKI, elevated liver enzymes, pulm edema) needs immediate action w/ IV drip meds like NTG, Na nitroprusside, Labetalol/ Esmolol, Nicardipine & fenoldopam. PO meds can also be used like Hydralazin &/or Clonidine while waiting for the drip.
- **HTN urgency** (same as emergency but no end organ damage) can be managed on the floor w/ PO agents like nitropaste (topical), hydralazine, Clonidine, captopril (short acting NOT lisinopril which is long acting) & labetalol. Do NOT ↓ BP more than 25% in the 1st 6 hrs (could cause cerebral hypoperfusion). Non-compliance w/ HTN meds (especially Clonidine & β blocker) is a common reason for extreme HTN.
- **Elevated BP can be caused by CNS problems** like CVA or elevated intra-cranial pressure (ICP). Do NOT ↓ systolic BP <140s-150s in the 1st 1-2 days

46

- **Chronic NSAID** use causes/worsens HTN. Switch to Tylenol if possible.

> **Attention**: decongestants OTC that contain ephedrine could cause worsening HTN →HTN urgency/emergency. Always review new meds for worsening HTN.

- **Thiazides** ↑ serum Ca (& uric acid), whereas **furosemide** ↓ Ca.
- **Controlling BP is very essential** for systolic & diastolic CHF Tx (afterload reduction)
- ↓ **PO intake** is a problem for pt w/ HTN as most of the meds are PO & IV HTN meds is NOT recommended in the floor (mostly in the ICU). Clonidine patches are a good option.

9. Anticoagulation

Various drugs are used for anticoagx, known as 'blood thinners' in layman terminology. There are different indications & guidelines for each of them & therefore, each of them will be discussed separately.

Heparin:

Mechanism of action: activates anti-thrombin III, which inactivates clotting enzymes, such as thrombin & Factor Xa. Two major formulations of heparin are unfractionated heparin (UFH) & low-molecular weight heparin (LMWH). LMWH mainly acts by inactivating factor Xa.

Uses: Heparin & its other formulations are used for treating venous thromboembolism (VTE), which includes both deep vein thrombosis (DVT) & pulm embolism. Guidelines recommend treating any episode of VTE w/ 4-5 days of either UFH heparin (IV heparin drip) or LMWH like Enoxaparin (subcutaneous injection), while "bridging" w/ Coumadin to maintain therapeutic INR for at least 2 days before discharge.
For UFH (IV drip), there is a weight-based heparin dosing protocol (nurses usually manage it by a protocol). Therefore, the pt has to be admitted to the hospital. LMWH also has a weight-based dosing. However, it is a subcutaneous injection & so pts can be discharged on it.

LMWH is contraindicated in pts w/ renal insufficiency: avoid in ESR & requires dose adjustments in pts w/ eGFR <30 (once daily instead of twice daily dosing). Heparin (subcutaneous) & LMWH (at lower doses) are also used as prophylaxis to prevent episodes of VTE in immobilized pts, including pts lying in hospital beds for long periods of time.

Adverse effects: Heparin-induced thrombocytopenia (HIT) can develop w/ any dose or type of heparin, & is of two types. Type 1 is a non-immune mediated process

48

where the decline in platelet count is w/ in the first 24-48 hrs, & does NOT require stopping heparin. Type 2 is an immune-mediated process where the decline in platelet count occurs between 5-14 days, & requires stopping all forms of heparin. Type 2 may require Tx w/ argatroban due to high risk of associated arterial or venous thrombosis. Other adverse effects include hyperkalemia & osteoporosis.

Warfarin:

Mechanism of action: acts by inhibiting vitamin-K dependent pro-coagulant factors, namely factors II, VII, IX, X & anti-coagulant factors, protein C & S synthesized by the liver. It takes about 5 days to achieve full anti-coagulant effect. Initially, due to rapid depletion of Protein C before the other pro-coagulant factors, there is a risk of hypercoagulability & warfarin-induced skin necrosis. Therefore, heparin therapy should be used in the first 2-3days of anticoagx, along w/ Coumadin (bridging therapy). When beginning Warfarin, INR needs to be checked w/ in the first week to make dosage adjustments, then carefully monitored monthly. Also, you have to consider the dangers of using Warfarin in an elderly pt at risk for falls (weigh risks & benefits w/ the pt or his/her family).

Uses:

Tx of VTE: After about 5 days of heparin, an episode of DVT or pulm embolism requires long-term Tx w/ an PO anti-coagulant for several months. Duration depends on risk of recurrent VTE & bleeding – first episode of VTE w/ reversible factors such as immobilization due to trauma, surgery, PO contraceptive pills, & long-duration air travel requires Tx for 3 months. Pts w/ cancer should receive anticoagx until cancer resolves. Pts w/ inherited hypercoagulable states, such as Factor V Leiden, or Protein C, S or ATIII deficiencies usually require Tx for over 6 months. If a pt has recurrent idiopathic VTE, they require anticoagx for life unless contraindications such hemorrhage develops.

Anticoagx for artificial heart valves: Target INR depends on the type of heart valve used. For any tissue valve at any location, target INR is between 2-3 for 3 months & then lifelong ASA. If a mechanical (metal) valve is placed, pt will mostly need lifelong Coumadin (depends on the valve location mitral/aortic & the type St. Jude's or others).

Anticoagx for a fib: People w/ A fib are at an↑ risk for stroke. A CHADS2 score is a simple pneumonic to help assess the risk of stroke in a pt w/ non-rheumatic a fib. CHADS2 stands for **Congestive** heart Failure (1 point), **HTN** (1 point), **Age** ≥75 years (1 point), **D**iabetes mellitus (1 point), & prior hx of **S**troke or TIA (**2** points, hence the 2 by the S). Generally, a score of 2 or above is considered a strong indication for anticoagx.

CHA2DS2VASc scoring system is more accurate tool **(use if CHADS2 score is 0 or 1)** to assess the need for anticoagx (especially elderly women). It stands for CHF (1 point), HTN (1 point), Age ≥ 75 (2 points), DM (1 point), Stroke (2 points), Vascular disease (1 point), Age 65-74 (1 point), Sex (Sex category w/ 1 point if female). Female w/ a score of ≥ 2 needs to be considered for long-term anticoagx (or male ≥ 1).

How to reverse a high INR from Coumadin overdose: For asymptomatic minor INR elevations (INR <5), no intervention is needed other than holding Coumadin & then restarting it at a lower dose once INR is in target range. For an INR between 5-9 (w/o bleeding), hold all anti-thrombotic therapy, & repeat INR again the next day. If the INR is still rising or there is a high risk of bleeding, give vitamin K PO (usually, a low dose such as 1mg is preferred).

If the **INR is >9 (w/o bleeding),** give vitamin K (2-10 mg PO) & repeat the INR in 24-28 hrs. Repeat the vitamin K dose as needed (needs hours to days to work).

If there is a **minor bleed w/ any INR level**, vitamin K 1-5 mg PO or IV must be given. Recheck INR in 24 hrs & if it still NOT controlled, repeat the vitamin K dosage. If bleeding still persists after repeat vitamin K, it must be treated as a major bleed.

Any **major bleeding** for a pt on Coumadin should be treated w/ vitamin K IV 10 mg over 10-20 minutes & FFP (rechecked INR in 6-12 hrs) & continue vitamin K & FFP until bleeding has stopped. Surgical intervention to stop the bleeding may also be considered.

Anticoagx after coronary artery stenting: Current guidelines recommend anticoagx w/ dual anti-platelet therapy (DAPT), which includes ASA w/ either clopidogrel (most commonly used) or others such as prasugrel, ticagrelor, or ticlopidine. Duration of therapy for both drug-eluting stents (DES) & bare metal stents (BMS) is 12 months. Minimum duration of uninterrupted therapy is 4 weeks for BMS, & 6 months for DES (every effort to continue therapy should be made prior to stopping at this early duration). Sometimes for repeated stenting & extensive CAD, Plavix & ASA should be considered for life if NOT contraindicated (e.g., tendency to bleed)

Novel PO anticoagulants: Dabigatran (Pradaxa), apixaban (Eliquis), & rivaroxaban (Xarelto) are novel PO anticoagulants that can be used as alternatives to warfarin in certain circumstances, such as in non-valvular a fib stroke prevention. These have an advantage in that there is no need to monitor INR, & there is ↓ risk of bleeding, especially w/ apixaban & rivaroxaban. However, in the event of a major bleed, there are still no reversal agents for these new agents, as is the case w/ warfarin. They are associated w/ ↓ risk of major bleeding episodes such as intra-cranial bleeds, but have high risk of GI bleeds. Usually they are expensive & some insurance companies do NOT cover them.

Special consideration:

- **Heparin IV drip is preferred for critically ill pts or those expected to have surgical intervention** (e.g., CABG or heart catheterization) due to the quick wash off period (short half-life; 4-6hours). LMWH has longer half-life of 12-24 hrs. So "bridging" from oral anticoagx like warfarin to IV heparin drip is necessary by holding the warfarin & monitoring INR daily. Start heparin drip when INR is subtherapeutic (<2 or 2.5).

Attention: Do NOT stop heparin drip unless the procedure/surgery is confirmed & resume heparin ASAP simultaneously w/ warfarin until INR is therapeutic. Successful "bridging" is important especially for pts with mechanical valves.

- **Pts on anticoagx (like warfarin) who presented w/ bleeding (usually from GI tract):** INR should be checked & may be reversed as indicated above, considering the INR level & severity of the bleed. Consider resuming warfarin after Tx (e.g., clipping or cauterizing a bleeding source EGD & colonoscopy) & you may need to discuss risk & benefits of resuming anticoagx meds w/ the pt in case of recurrence.
- **Facts about Plavix:**
  A. Need to be stopped five days before any non-emergent surgery (e.g., CABG) to be "washed out" & ↓ the bleeding risk.
  B. Hold off giving plavix at the time of chest pain presentation for pts who may need CABG after the heart cath (like elderly w/ DM or ESRD on HD). Plavix can be given at the time of the heart cath if stent/s are indicated.

C. All efforts should be made to keep Plavix for at least 6months s/p DES & 6weeks s/p BMS to prevent in-stent stenosis (try to postpone any elective surgeries until after these dates).

- **Triple oral antithrombotic therapy (TOAT)** is needed sometimes for cardiovascular disease. It means the concomitant use of dual antiplatelet therapy (DAPT) w/ aspirin & ADP platelet receptor blocker like Plavix or Effient (as s/p DUS) & oral anticoagulation (OAC) like after A fib diagnosis w/ high CHADS2 score ($\geq$ 2). All efforts should be made to stop any of them when they are NOT indicated anymore due to the high bleeding risk (stop plavix after 1 yr of DUS). INR should be monitored more frequently (target INR is different in TOAT, metal valve: 2. 5-3, a fib: 2-2. 5).

- **Screening for thrombophilia & malignancy following a first episode of unprovoked venothrombotic event (VTE) is controversial.** Limited cancer screening is acceptable for the 1st episode of idiopathic VTE (i.e., no CT/PET scans) with a clinical evaluation (focused malignancy hx like weight loss, $\downarrow$ appetite, SOB, constipation or hematuria), basic laboratory testing (like CBC, CMP, & ESR), age-appropriate cancer screening (like mammogram, & colonoscopy as indicated) & CXR (& following the abnormal results w/ full work up). More extensive cancer screening strategies are NOT justified in this population but may be warranted for higher cancer risk pts (like recurrent VTE despite anticoagx & hepatic or portal vein thrombosis).
  If you decided to go with the extensive thrombophilia work up (like after the 2nd VTE), **postpone the tests for few weeks** (mostly as an out pt) after the even as the clotting even & the anticoagx meds will affect the tests results. Factor V Leiden, prothrombin gene mutation,

antiphosphospholipid antibodies, factor C & S deficiency are prothrombogenic factors. Surgery (especially orthopedics), pregnancy, oral contraceptives, immobilization, CHF, & central lines are common acquired etiology as well.

- **Prophylactic anticoagulation:** is very important to prevent DVT/PE in certain populations in addition to the in pt DVT prophylaxis (heparin 5000 u TID or LMWH like Daltiparin –better- or Lovenox). Pts w/ fractures, immobile, or cancer may need 3-6 months of lovenox (preferred for oncology pts) or oral anticoagx agents. Clinical trials support that prophylaxis & showing good mortality benefits but guidelines is still NOT totally supporting it, yet (consult hematology PRN). IVC filter is a controversial option to prevent PE (commonly it is indicated to prevent 2nd PE in pts with known DVT who had 1st PE & failed anticoagx).

10. Nausea & vomiting (N/V)

Very common Sx. There is a vast majority of causes such as meds, chemo, underlying illness, reflux, etc. Always evaluate the pt at the bedside for new-onset vomiting or abdominal pain, persistent vomiting, or hematemesis. For symptomatic control, you can give the pt an antiemetic from the list below.

Medication

- **Ondansetron (Zofran):** serotonin 5-HT3 receptor antagonist. Very commonly used for any N/V w/ minimum side effect (prolong QT). Specific for cancer pts (chemo/radiotherapy) & surgery (prevent & Tx N/V).
- **Prochlorperazine** (Compazine) PO/IV/IM. Selectively antagonizes dopamine D2 receptors. **Side effects** include urinary retention, HoTN, spastic torticollis, dystonia (treat w/ Benadryl or Benztropine), cytopenias, & QT prolongation
- **Metoclopramide** (Reglan) PO/IV. Antagonizes central & peripheral dopamine receptors. **Side effects** include extrapyramidal Sx, urinary frequency, cytopenias, SVT, HTN, & sedation
- **Promethazine** (Phenergan) PO/IM/PR (antihistamine→hwill also produce sedation). Antagonizes central & peripheral H1 receptors (non-selective antihistamine). **Side effects** include sedation, cytopenias, & urinary retention
- **Lorazepam** (Ativan) IV/PO. Binds to benzodiazepine receptors, enhances GABA effects. NOT commonly used to Tx N/V alone but can be considered if sedation is needed as well. **Side effects** include delirium in the elderly & sedation.
- **Chemotherapy-induced:** Consider using serotonin antagonists, such as **ondansetron (Zofran)** or, as a last resort, **Marinol** (Cannabis derivative, very expensive, & appetite stimulator),

which works on cannabinoid receptors in the brain & is a schedule III drug. It is approved for chemotherapy-induced N/V.

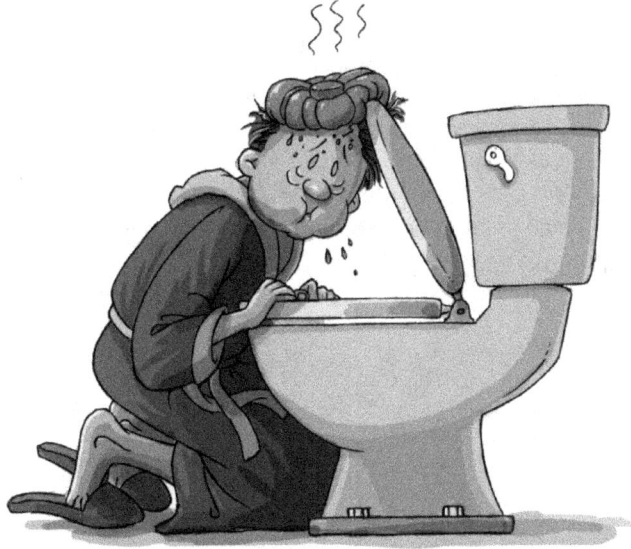

Nausea & vomiting are nonspecific Sx & can be very debilitating.

Special considerations

- **Fluid hydration:** If the pt canNOT tolerate PO, consider making the pt NPO & starting IV hydration along w/ PO/IV antiemetics (it is a reason for admission if N/V is refractory to PO antiemetics).

> **Attention**: Always ensure that the pt is hydrated & electrolytes are corrected.

- **Zofran has no sedating effect** (NOT dopamine antagonist) like Phenergan (1st generation antihistamine w/ antidopaminergic effect) &

Raglan (antidopaminergic effect w/ ↑ GI motility & lower esophageal tone)

- **Radiology:** If obstruction is a possible etiology, order an abdominal series x-ray. If there is evidence of an obstruction or ileus, place an NG Tube to help decompress the stomach
- **Usually NJ tube is for refractory N/V** pts to decompress the stomach for any etiology (NOT just obstruction).

Resolution: As the Sx resolve, slowly advance the diet from clear liquid to full liquid to soft mechanical to regular (as indicated).

11. Medicine facts (side effects, onset of side effects, & off-label therapeutic uses)

Common facts for common meds commonly used:

- **QT interval prolongation:** can be caused by a lot of meds like quinolones, antiarrhythmic meds (amiodarone/tykosin/procainamide), psychiatry meds (fluoxetine/quetiapine/haldol), pain meds (methadone), & a lot of others. This can evolve to torsades de pointes (TdP), which is a unique V tachycardia. Monitor QTc before & on a regular basis after starting & consider stopping the meds if QTc >500-550. Check K & Mg & replete as needed. Treat TdP w/ ↑ dose IV Mg along w/ ACLS.
- **Statins:** ↑ Creatine kinase (from muscles) & AST/ALT. Statins can help maintaining sinus rhythm after a fib cardioversion (ACE inhibitors can help as well maintaining sinus rhythm), but it is still NOT used for that purpose alone.
- **Pregnancy & antiemetics:** non-pharmacological methods are preferred like eating small meals, avoiding strong odors, getting enough sleep, & avoiding fatigue. Evidence is insufficient regarding the safety of most of the meds. Many class C antiemetic meds are prescribed during pregnancy when benefits> risks. **Meds:** multivitamins, Zofran, Phenergan, Reglan, & Meclizine.
- **Cirrhosis & Tylenol:** up to 2 g/day is safe (up to 4g/day in healthy person). Toxicity is when levels are up to 10-15 g/day. Acetylcysteine is the antidote.
- **Cirrhosis & increased Ammonia:** Use Lactulose (laxatives, monitor) & Rifaximine (abx). NO need to monitor Ammonia levels &

follow up clinical response (up titrate lactulose dose to target 3-4 bowel movements)
- **Pulmonary HTN & Remodulin (**peripheral prostacyclin vasodilator) infusion pump: do NOT hold because rebound pulm HTN may occur & could be catastrophic.
- **Metoprolol & Coreg for A fibTx:** both can rate control the heart. Coreg has alpha-1 blocking activity & can cause HoTN (metoprolol causes less HoTN). So choose coreg if you want to control HTN along w/ slowing the rate.

> **Attention:** max β blocker and ACEi doses for CHF pts before adding another CHF meds to get the mortality benefits (like 25bid for coreg and 40 for lisinopril).

- **Blood levels:** of some meds should be monitored to assure therapeutic levels & avoid toxicity. Check levels after starting new meds → change doses & /or start another med incase of drug-drug interaction. Examples: Vanc, Dilantin, Valproic acid, phenobarbital, tacrolimus, digoxin, lithium (some meds can cause the adverse effect even on therapeutic levels like brady or tachy arrhythmias w/ digoxin & lithium). Make sure you correct the phenytoin level for albumin in case of hypoalbuminemia (false low levels if albumin is low).
- **Nitroglycerin facts: 1.** NTG w/ Viagra can cause refractory HoTN. **2.** Do NOT give NTG if SBP is <90. **3.** NTG is used to relieve ischemic pain (up to 3 doses, 0. 4mg q5min), so no need for NTG if there is no pain. **4.** NTG is contraindicated for inferior MI since those pts are volume-dependent (actually sometime they require IV fluids to maintain BP). NTG will ↓ the preload which they will NOT tolerate (treat HoTN w/ IV fluids)

- **Changes in thyroxine** replacement therapy for hypothyroidism require 4-6 weeks to affect the TSH levels. Small changes in TSH in the in-pt setting do NOT require synthroid dose adjustments. **In general:** do NOT adjust thyroxine dose for pts in the hospital as TSH changes is maybe just from sick thyroid syndrome & may be misleading (repeat TSH in few weeks if abnormal).
- **Warfarin** is a common anticoagx medicine & requires continuous INR monitoring in warfarin clinic or, for selective pts, at home.
- **Morphines & narcotics (as well as benzodiazepines/sedatives in general)** can cause respiratory suppression for pts who already have underlying disorders like COPD & pulm fibrosis. Use w/ caution (avoid for pts w/ baseline hypoactive delirium to avoid intubation due to inability to protect airways).
- **PPI** (or H2 blocker) for GI & **heparin sq** for DVT prophylaxis are commonly used in the hospital pts. They are specifically important for ICU pts due to ↓ mobility & NPO status.

> **Attention**: to NOT start heparin on bleeding pt (like GI bleeding), while no real contraindication for PPI. May be PPI is NOT needed for pts admitted for observation for any reason if they are eating normally. PPI ↑ PNA risk.

- **Clonidine** is α1 agonist & is used for HTN. In the ICU, it can be used as a sedative agent (like Precedex but NOT commonly used for that purpose)
- **Clindamycin** can is strongly associated with C diff diarrhea but it can be a direct effect from the medicine itself, stop the medicine & test for C diff if diarrhea did NOT improve. It covers CA-

MRSA & it has anti-toxin quality (from toxin producing organism like strep) make it preferred for mild-moderate out or even in pt cellulitis Tx (small % of strep developed resistance to clindamycin; reassess & switch abx prn)

- **Bactrim** has K sparing ability in the kidney like sprinolactone & therefore can cause hyperkalemia.

> **Attention**: to hyperkalemia when Bactrim is used with other meds like ACEi & sprinolactone.

- **SSRI can cause SIADH** (hyponatremia w/o edema usually).
- **Loop diuretics & Na/ urine osmolarity:** although loop diuretics affect Na reabsorption (as thiazides); hyponatremia is less comparing to thiazides due to the higher urine osmolarity & Na concentration with thiazides (different mechanism of action). Maybe it is safe to assume that urine is hypertonic with thiazides & hypo or isotonic with loops. Ethacrynic acid is a loop diuretic but does NOT contain sulfa.
- **"Steroid taper":** usually prescribed for short period of time (like for COPD or Asthma) after giving moderate-high doses of steroids for >7-10 days (moderate-high prednisone dose is ≥20mg/day) to prevent pituitary-adrenal axis suppression. No need for that taper if the steroid dose is small (like 5 mg prednisone daily) or the high dose is <7days. No specific guidelines for steroid taper & it is mostly provider dependent.

Example: Prednisone 60mg for 3 days, 40mg for 3 days, 20mg for 3days, 10mg for 3 days & 5mg for 3 days & then stop. "Steroid taper" can be indicated also for different reason as a part of the therapy like to prevent frequent COPD exacerbations.

- **Common steroids comparison (w/doses)**

Hydrocortisone	Prednisone	Dexamethasone
20mg equal to	5mg equal to	1mg
High mineral & low anti-inflammatory activity (good for shock).	Medium mineral & medium anti-inflammatory activity	Low mineral & high anti-inflammatory activity (good for Cancer).

- **Pyridium:** is urinary analgesic for UTI, changes urine color normally to red/orange (inform the pt), use for short period (<2-3 days), avoid in case of AKI/CKD.

- **Antipsychotics:** used for positive Sx like delirium, psychosis (schizophrenia or mania) or negative Sx like flat affect or social withdrawal. 1st Gen. like Haldol has antidopamine effect & it is safer for elderly (w/ dementia) & cardiac pts while 2nd Gen. are antidopamine & serotonin (& anticholinergic as a side-effect) like Olanzapine ($\uparrow$ appetite & $\uparrow$ blood sugar) /Seroquel ($\uparrow$ appetite & help sleeping)/Abilify ($\downarrow$ appetite & least anticholinergic)/Clozapine (cause agranulocytosis & used after 2 other antipsychotic fail). Both have the same antipsychotic effect but 2nd gen. help in negative Sx (unlike 1st Gen.). Look for the long acting forms (injections) when adherence is a problem.

- **Estrogen & Desmopressin (DDAVP):** help in improving coagulation in case of bleeding disorders like in liver disease. DDAVP $\uparrow$ Von willebrand factor release from endothelial cells. Use **Fibrin spray (Tisseel)** for superficial bleeding due to hemostatic effect.

- **Atropine:** can be indicated in symptomatic bradycardias like in heart blocks & it works by ↓ the parasympathic pathway → ↑ sympathic pathway. Due to the special heart innervation system (atriums→ parasympathic & sympathic but ventricles→just sympathic), atropine (works on parasympathic) may NOT work if the AV node is NOT conducting (consider pacemaker).
- **Always check** if any medicine you will prescribe needs to be **renally dosed** in case of AKI/CKD/ESRD. Do the same with Cirrhosis pts.
- **Allergic cross-reactivity:** angioedema from ACEi has ≈ 10% risk of allergy w/ ARBs & also anaphylactic from penicillin has ≈ 10% risk of allergy w/ cephalosporin & ≈ 1% w/ Aztreonam.

12. Outpatient Medicine

Important part of residency & it can be a future career. The following are some common pathology you may encounter in the clinic (Many others are included elsewhere in detail throughout the book).

Lipids: New guidelines for Tx are NOT totally depending on the actual lipid blood levels
- Start **high potency** statins on
  1. Individuals w/ clinical atherosclerotic cardiovascular disease (like CAD or CVA)
  2. Individuals w/ LDL-cholesterol levels $\geq$190.

- Start **moderate potency** statins on:
  1. Individuals w/ diabetes aged 40 to 75 years old w/ LDL-cholesterol levels between 70 & 189 mg/dL & w/o evidence of atherosclerotic cardiovascular disease.
  2. Individuals w/o evidence of cardiovascular disease or diabetes but who have LDL-cholesterol levels between 70 & 189 mg/dL & a 10-year risk of atherosclerotic cardiovascular disease (ASCVD calculator is available online)$\geq$ 7. 5% (you can use high potency as well instead of moderate).

Statins:
High potency: Atorvastatin 40-80mg & Rosuvastatins 20-40mg (the goal is to achieve at least a 50% reduction in LDL).
Moderate potency: The rest of statins (like Simvastatins) including the high potency at lower doses (lowers LDL cholesterol 30% to 49%). Follow-up the lipid panel in 8-12 weeks after starting therapy & yearly afterwards. Get LFT as a baseline before therapy & another one in 3 months (acceptable to have elevated AST/ALT up to 3 times of normal limits). There is no need to repeat LFT unless clinically indicated (RUQ pain, ictrus, itching, etc).

Ostoartheritis (OA): Common, usually in the knees & cervical vertebrae. X-ray is a good initial test & usually the severity of the arthritis does NOT necessarily correlate w/ the severity of the Sx (mild arthritis could cause severe Sx & vice versa). Start Tylenol & NSAIDs if NOT contraindicated (CHF, GI bleeding, CKD, bleeding tendency, etc) & reevaluate. Consider further testing like MRI/CT scan if you expect a surgical intervention & refer to orthopedics. Usually stiffness from OA lasts<30minuts (Rheumatoid arthritis RA lasts>30m & has +RF, +CCP)

Lower back pain (LBP): #1 disability etiology in US for pts <40 yo. Acute <6 weeks while chronic >3 months. R/o serious diagnosis (need urgent referral to neurosurgery) like **Cauda Equina Syndrome** (ask about incontinence & saddle paresthesia & motor or sensory impairment) & **spinal stenosis** (pain on walking which relieved by rest →pseudoclaudication).
Hx & physical exam is essential to r/o **radical neuropathies** (pain radiating down the leg in a dermatome way, sensory & strength exam, including walking on toes & heals is warranted to localize the nerve involvement, L5/S1). **Muscle spasm** pain is very common (trauma or heavy lifting/exercising) which is usually very severe, sudden & disabling.
Tests: Imaging studies (CT or MRI are better than plan X-rays) in the first 4-6 weeks are not necessary unless **alarming Sx** present like hx of cancer (mets), illicit injection drugs (osteomyelitis or abscess), major neurologic deficits (disk problem), rest pain, systemic Sx like fever, & prolonged steroids use. Note that disk protrusion/heraniation ≠ back pain as bulging discs are seen in more than 50 percent of asymptomatic patients; asymptomatic herniated discs are seen as well, though less frequently.

Tx: pain meds as indicated in the pain meds ladder: Tylenol, NSAIDs, lortab, oxycodone, PO or IV morphine or dilaudid (for 1 month/no need for bed-rest/encourage exercise as tolerated). Know what meds that pt is taking at home & resume them as indicated (for hospital pts). **Consider high dose steroid** (Solu-Medrol IV) for spinal compression Sx & stat neurosurgery consult (or refer to them the chronic debilitating cases if the pt is willing surgery). **Conisder chiropractor & physical therapy** (for another 1 month if pain persist >1 month on pain meds). Refer to neurosurgery or neurology after 2 months of conservative Tx with pain meds & physical therapy. **Consider Psychological distress or secondary gains** for chronic LBP w/ "inappropriate pain" signs. Neck pain is very similar to LBP in management.

Infection:
- **URI:** presents w/ cough (may be w/ green/yellow sputum which does NOT necessarily means bacterial infx but could be viral), fever, & dyspnea. Viral mostly associated w/ runny nose, sneezing, conjunctivitis, sick contact & pt does NOT look very sick (viral is self-limited & treat supportively w/ 1st G antihistamine, cough meds, etc). If bacterial: Azithromycin (z pack) is a good option.
- **Pharyngitis/tonsillitis/sinusitis**: viral or bacterial. **CENTOR criteria**: can guide to start abx (mainly used for pharyngitis); as it is hard to differentiate between viral vs bacterial infx by just physical exam or radiology.

Ask about 4 things:
Fever>38c, cervical adenopathy, tonsillar exudates, & the absent of cough or rhinitis (calculator **available online**).

If **0-1** present→ **no abx**
2-3 → **rapid strep** swab test & if positive→ start abx (z pack or Augmentin),
4→ **start abx** w/o further testing.

Palpate for sinus tenderness & do trans-illumination test of maxillary sinus (properly trans-illuminated in case of air→ normal; trans illumination is NOT equal on both sides→ sinusitis).

- **UTI:** if lower (suprapubic tenderness, dysuria, frequency) order urine analysis & start abx (like bactrim or Ciprofloxacin for 3 days if uncomplicated), if upper UTI (fever, chills, CVA tenderness, dysuria) order UA & assess the need for hospital admission (elderly, multiple comorbidities, septic signs, etc) for IV abx (Ciprofloxacin or zosyn). UTI can be categorized to "uncomplicated", which is in lower UTI in female for the 1st time. The rest is complicated (male even for the 1st time, recurrence, Upper UTI, etc).

Attention: no need to follow UTI response to abx by urine analysis or urine Cx. Clinical improvement is enough (unless in pregnancy → Tx even asymptomatic bacteriuria and assure resolution w/ negative urine Cx)

Gout: Usually affects the big toe (Podagra) & other joints. NO need to confirm diagnoses by arthrocentesis (to see the monosodium urate crystals).
Clinical diagnosis is enough, unless you consider another diagnose like septic joint (WBC>2k in gout while >50k in septic joint w/ positive stain & culture).
 Tx of choice: NSAIDs (if NOT contraindicated like in CKD), then colchicine, local steroid injection, & lastly systemic steroids (like prednisone PO). **Continue allopurinol if pt was on it before the flare, but do NOT initiate it** in the acute attack (rapid up or down changes in uric acid blood levels may worsen gouty attack). Scheduled dose of daily colchicines for maintenance (not just on the acute flare) can also be prescribed in case of allopurinol allergy (should be

dosed renally). **Probenecid** (inhipit uric acid tubular reabsorption but contraindicated in CKD) & **Uloric** (like allopurinol but expensive). Target uric acid <7.

Smoke/EtOH & illicit drugs: assess for abuse in every visit & counsel to stop w/ a clear direct sentence like "this abuse will/already hurt your body & vital organs like lung, heart, liver, etc & if you stop you may stop the progression. If you are interested I can assist you". If the pt is NOT interested, you can readdress it in a later visit (spending much time in counseling if the pt is NOT interested in quitting did NOT prove to be successful). Offer nicotine patches/gum or even meds like Wellbutrin & Chantix (good for depression as well) to ↓ grieving Sx (but insurance may NOT cover them) or even referral to rehabilitation center (for EtOH & drug abuse)

Dermatology:
- **Shingles:** Reactivation of latent varicella-zoster virus (VZV) infx w/ in the sensory ganglia results in herpes zoster or "shingles". This syndrome is usually characterized by a painful, unilateral vesicular eruption in a dermatomal distribution. Early antiviral therapy (acyclovir for 1 week for age >50) can promote rapid healing of skin lesions, lessen the severity & duration of pain associated w/ acute neuritis, & reduces the incidence or severity of chronic pain.
- **Itching:** it can be from systemic disease like liver or renal disease. Allergy from new meds is a possible cause (try to stop new meds & monitor). Xerosis (dry skin) is a common cause for pruritus. Ask about excessive h & washing or may be new detergent (which can be contact dermatitis, could be treated w/ topical steroids).
  Tx: Moisturizers such as petrolatum can help the dry skin.
  Scabies: is another possible itching etiology, which usually presents w/ severe itching, often worse at night, & nondescript erythematous

papules. Family involvement strongly suggests the diagnosis.

Tx: Ivermectine PO (which can treat lice too) & /or Permethrin (Tx the family also & wash the linens).

Polypharmacy: Frequent routine review to verify need for meds & appropriate dosing is an important aspect of optimal pt (especially elderly) care.

Altered mental status is a common adverse effect to polypharmacy (mostly psychiatry & pain meds). Assess risks & benefits for meds & consider stopping any med that has the same side effect (like statins, fibrates, & Niacins which may all damage the liver). Consider stopping meds that are NOT indicated any more like prophylactic statins for very elderly pts or anticoagx for elderly w/ ↑ risk of falls (after discussing risks & benefits).

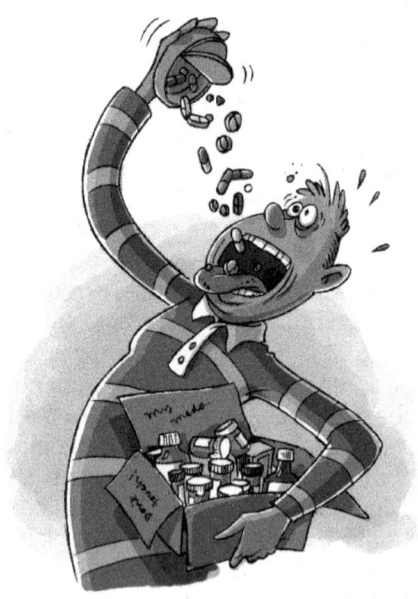

Polypharmacy is a common reason for AMS & meds interaction should be considered, especially for the elderly.

Heath Care Maintenance: In a general medicine clinic it's helpful to conclude each note w/ a health care maintenance section. This includes age & sex specific screening tests as well as vaccinations that are otherwise easy to overlook. **Common Vaccines & screening tests:**

- **PAP smear:** starting age 21-65 or 3 years after 1st sexual activity, q3 years (or q5years if PAP + HPV test). Optimal frequency is NOT established (q1-2 years is acceptable)
- **Mammogram:** females >50 usually or age 40-50 if the pt wants (usually every 1-2 years).
- **AAA screen w/ abdominal US:** male age 65-75 if ever smoker
- **Colonoscopy:** any pt >50, every 10 years (or FOBT + flex sig q5years)
- **Lung cancer screen w/ chest CT scan:** age 55-80 q1 year if >30 pack years, current smoker, or quit w/ in last 15 years (do NOT screen if quit>15 years)
- **Hyperlipidemia:** male>35 & female >45, q5 years.
- **PSA:** any male >50 (if the pt agrees but generally NOT recommended for screening w/o risks). Refer to GU for biopsy if PSA>7 (rectal exam is NOT recommended for screening)
- **DEXA scan for osteoporosis:** female >65 or <65 w/ fracture, q 2-8 years.
- **Vaccines:**
Influenza: yearly for all adults.
Pneumovaccines: pneumococcal polysaccharide vaccine (PPSV23), elderly>65, DM, CHF, CKD, Asthma/COPD, asplenic pts, & others.

> **Attention**: Usually screening tests are NOT recommended for pt >75 yo or pts w/ life expectancy <10 years (physician dependent).

Zoster: > 60 yo, one time (life attenuated).
Other life attenuated vaccines: Varicella, MMR, yellow fever, oral polio, & Nasal flu (most of the others are inactivated).
Tdap/Td: >19 yo, one time (but tetanus q10 yrs)
HPV vaccine: all male & female age 13-26 yo.

13. Electrolyte imbalances

Hypernatremia

This always implies a free water deficit. It leads to neurological abnormalities, such as confusion, disorientation, seizure or even coma. Severity of Sx may vary depending on the chronicity of the hyponatremia.

Causes:
1. **Hypovolemia with Dehydration,** which is water loss more than Na (poor PO intake, diarrhea, DKA, elderly w/ AMS, fever, PNA or other types of insensible losses). Hypovolemia is different than dehydration due to the equal loss of water & Na in the former.
Tx is w/ volume expansion & fluid replacement. Rate of correction depends on the duration of hypernatremia.
2. **Normo- or hypervolemia hypernatremia,** such as **Diabetes Insipidus (DI):** There are two types: central & nephrogenic. Both give the following: ↓urine osmolality, & ↑ urine volume.
a) Central DI is caused by a failure to produce antidiuretic hormone (ADH) in the brain. The pt will have a prompt ↑ in urine osmolarity w/ administration of DDAVP. Tx is w/ DDAVP (vasopressin).
b) Nephrogenic DI is caused by insensitivity of the kidney to ADH. Pt will have no change in both urine volume & osmolarity w/ DDAVP.

Tx is to correct the underlying cause (e.g. hypokalemia, hypercalcemia). Use thiazide diuretics for other causes.

Hyponatremia:

Hypo-osmolar (True) Hyponatremia
May present (similar to hypernatremia) w/ neurologic abnormalities, such as confusion, disorientation, seizures, or coma. The first step in management is to

assess volume status to determine the cause, & therefore, the Tx.

1. **Hypervolemic hyponatremia:** Pts w/ edema & swelling. Causes: Congestive heart failure (CHF), Nephrotic syndrome or Cirrhosis. Tx is to correct the underlying cause (& usually fluid restriction to <800cc/day). For CHF pts, hyponatremia is a prognostic marker for disease progression & usually does NOT need to be treated if it is asymptomatic & NOT severe (>120meq/L).

Tx: loop diuretics & optimize CHF meds to improve heart function (in CHF). Consider Albumin infusion (in cirrhosis).

2. **Hypovolemic hyponatremia: Causes:** Volume depletion (due to diuretics, vomiting, & diarrhea) **causes an appropriate ADH response** →↑ water retention & Na level ↓. **Tx** is by correcting the underlying cause & normal saline replacement (to correct the volume & remove ADH stimulation). Remember to check serum Na frequently during replacement.

3. **Euvolemic hyponatremia:**
Causes:
- **SIADH (Syndrome of Inappropriate ADH):** usually due to CNS problem or malignancy like small cell carcinoma in the lung. No volume deficits in SIADH. Tests: ↑ urine Na (>20 mEq/L), ↑ urine osmolality (>100 mOsm/Kg), ↓ serum osmolality (<290 mOsm/Kg), Normal Cr, BUN & Bicarbonate
- **Addison's disease** (insufficient aldosterone production): The key to this diagnosis is the presence of hyponatremia w/ **hyperkalemia & mild metabolic acidosis along w/ HoTN.** Treat w/ aldosterone replacement (fludrocortisone).
- **Hypothyroidism, psychogenic polydipsia, & hyperglycemia (**artificial "pseudo" drop in Na)

Tx:

- If mild or no Sx, treat by restricting fluids & managing the underlying problem.
- If moderate to severe or neurologic Sx, treat w/ the following: NS infusion w/ loop diuretics or Hypertonic 3% saline (which ↑ Na by 10meq/L for every one liter)
- Check serum Na frequently. Do NOT correct serum Na more than 10-12 mEq/L in the first 24 hrs. Correction rate can go up to 4-6meq/L in the first 6 hrs if severe Sx like seizure is present. Quick correction can cause permanent pontine osmotic demyelination & paralysis
- ADH blockers (conivaptan & tolvaptan) for refractory cases.

Hyperkalemia:
Common causes:

- Renal failure (prevents K excretion) w/ ↑ K diet or missing dialysis (for ESRD pts)
- Metabolic acidosis (↓ renal K excretion & transcellular shift out of the cells) & insulin deficiency, such as DKA
- Medicine: like K-sparing diuretics (such as spironolactone), digoxin toxicity, ACE inhibitors & ARBs (inhibit aldosterone), & β blockers (while β-agonists help in decreasing K; albuterol inhaler can be used for hyperkalemia)
- ↑ release from tissues such as muscles (e.g. rhabdomyolysis) or red blood cells (e.g. hemolysis).
- Adrenal aldosterone deficiency (Addison's disease), so check BP for HoTN
- Type IV renal Tubular Acidosis RTA (↓ aldosterone effect)
- Pseudohyperkalemia can occur for various reasons most commonly is delay in processing the blood sample (hemolysis). Repeat blood test if you suspect hemolysis.

Management: First, you have to order EKG & look for peaked T-waves & cardiac arrhythmias.
Severe hyperkalemia or hyperkalemia w/ EKG abnormalities: such as peaked T waves, administer Ca gluconate IV (to protect the heart), & then administer regular insulin (10 u IV)& glucose (50% dextrose IV, 50ml) or Albuterol (nebulizer) to shift K into the cells. Along w/ addressing the underlying problem like stopping the offending meds, treat DKA, get dialysis, etc. **Mild-Moderate hyperkalemia** (no EKG abnormalities), administer regular insulin, glucose (dextrose IV), & PO Kayexalate (to remove K from the body). Loop diuretics if pt makes urine. Correct causes for acidosis, rhabdomyolysis, & hemolysis. Bicarb is NOT very effective (do NOT use).

Hypokalemia:
Causes:
- Dietary insufficiency
- Diuretics (urinary loss)
- ↑ aldosterone (Conn's syndrome), causes HTN as well
- Vomiting (leads to metabolic alkalosis, which shifts K intracellularly, & volume depletion which ↑ aldosterone)
- Proximal (Type II) & distal (Type I) RTA
- Bartter syndrome (the defect here is similar to loop diuretics' mechanism) & Gitelman syndrome (similar to thiazide diuretics' mechanism)

Management: K replacement either PO or IV. Maybe both are needed especially in case of EKG changes (T wave flattening or any new arrhythmias) or severe hypokalemia. There is no maximum rate on PO K replacement, but IV K replacement must be slow so as to prevent an arrhythmia from overly rapid administration (peripheral 10mEq/hr, central 20mEq/hr). IV K also could be very vein irritating (burning sensation especially if small veins).

> **Attention:** Hypokalemia leads to cardiac rhythm disturbances (EKG can show "U-waves"), & it can also cause muscular weakness. This effect can be so severe that can cause rhabdomyolysis.

Hypomagnesaemia:
This presents w/ hypocalcaemia (Mg is required for PTH release), hypokalemia & cardiac arrhythmias.

Causes: Loop diuretics, alcohol abuse & drugs.

Tx: PO (GI irritation) or IV replacement depends on the severity.

Hypercalcemia:
Causes: The most common cause is primary hyperparathyroidism. Other causes include malignancy (PTHrP), granulomatous diseases (activate vitamin D), vitamin A & D intoxication, thiazide diuretics, tuberculosis, histoplasmosis, & berylliosis. Order malignancy work up for unexplained hypercalcemia.

Primary hyperparathyroidism: Most pts present w/ asymptomatic hypercalcemia. They may present w/ kidney stones, osteoporosis, osteomalacia, fractures, confusion, depression, constipation & abdominal pain. Labs show ↑ PTH & Ca. Tx is surgical removal in the following circumstances: any Symptomatic disease, renal insufficiency, markedly elevated 24-hr urine Ca or very elevated serum Ca (>12. 5)

Acute, severe hypercalcemia: The pt may present w/ confusion, constipation, nephrogenic DI (polyuria &

polydipsia), short QT syndrome on EKG, renal insufficiency, ATN & kidney stones.

Management:
1. Hydration: ↑ volume of normal saline, about 3-4 liters
2. Calcitonin (Miacalcin): 4IV/kg q12 hrs & repeat PRN (usually acts fast)
3. Bisphosphonate IV (pamidronate) especially for cancer related ↑ Ca (very potent but slow acting 2-4days) **4.Steroids** if the etiology is granulomatous disease. **Furosemide** is discouraged & should NOT be used even though it can ↓ Ca.

Hypocalcaemia:
Causes: Surgical removal of the parathyroid gland, hypomagnesaemia (Mg is required for PTH release) Vitamin D deficiency, acute hyperphosphatemia (phosphate binds Ca & lowers it), fat malabsorption (fat binds Ca in the gut & prevents absorption), PTH resistance: pseudohypoparathyroidism that accompanies a short fourth finger, round face, & mental retardation.

Presentation & management: Severe hypocalcemia presents w/ seizures, neural twitching (Chvostek's sign & Trousseau's sign), & arrhythmia (prolonged QT on EKG). Replace Ca IV (Ca gluconate 1-2 gr IV) or PO (CaCo$_3$ = TUMS) depending on severity. Treat the underlying problem (phosphate binder like Renagel for hyperphosphatemia, pancreatic enzymes for fat malabsorption in case of chronic pancreatitis, etc). Give activated Vitamin D for ESRD pts (like Calcitriol)

Special considerations:
- **Hypomagnesemia** can cause renal loss of K & "refractory" hypokalemia. Replete both electrolytes Mg & K together (in addition to the Ca as it also interferes w/ their levels in case of deficiency).

- **During Tx of DKA** you should replenish K even though it is normal. DKA management protocol from American Diabetes Association states that if K level is between 3. 3-5.3 give 20-30 mEq in each liter of IV fluid to keep serum K between 4 & 5 mEq/L.
- **Each 10 mEq K you give, total serum K will** ↑**by 0. 1 mEq/L** (IV replace the same as oral).
- **In case of hypocalcemia, check albumin level.** Total Ca concentration will change in parallel to the albumin concentration (because part of the Ca is bound to albumin). In general, the serum Ca concentration falls by 0. 8 mg/dL (0. 2 mmol/L) for every 1. 0 g/dL (10 g/L) fall in the serum albumin concentration (less than 4. 0 g/L). Ionized Ca does NOT need albumin correction (more expensive test usually ordered in critical pts & Symptomatic hypocalcemia)
- **Online calculator for free water deficits for hypernatremia** (depends on body weight, Na level, gender, etc) can calculate how much total free water you need to give. Usually D5 w/ ½ or ¼ NS is preferred for IV correction or free water flushes through NG or PEG tube.
- **Caution w/ quick correction of hypernatremia** (cerebral edema), especially if NOT Symptomatic (safe correction rate is 10 meq/L in 24hrs). Check Na level in 4-6 hrs from the time fluids are started & adjust the fluid rate as needed (check other electrolytes as well & correct as needed)
- **Hyperphosphatemia is common in CKD/ESRD pts.** Tx w/ either Ca-based binder like Ca acetate or non-Ca binder like Renagel (if hypercalcemia is an issue). Ca x PhO4 product >55 ↑ the probability for metastatic calcification in pts w/ ESRD & contribute to substantial amount of morbidity & mortality (recognize & treat early w/ phosphate binder).

.14. Miscellaneous:

A. Common cough meds

1. **Tylenol #3:** controlled meds (w/ codeine; suppress cough centrally)
2. **Robitussin (Guaifenesin):** Treats cough that is caused by colds, flu, or other conditions (expectorant that loosens mucus in lungs)
3. **Robitussin DM:** which is Robitussin plus Dextromethorphan (cough suppressant, act centrally in the medulla like codeine). You can include **Phenylephrine** as decongestant (vasoconstrictor) for URI (symptomatic relief)

> **Attention:** Do NOT "pseudo" treat the cough w/o treating the etiology (if possible).

B. Chronic management for asthma

- Start w/ short acting bronchodilator **(albuterol) prn** as rescue meds (for mild Asthma; 1st line Tx).
- If NOT controlled, add a chronic controller meds such as an **inhaled steroid (low dose** or you can step up to **moderate dose** for better control). You can start w/ controller +rescue meds prn if asthma is moderate or severe
- If inhaled albuterol prn & inhaled steroids moderate dose did NOT control Sx (pt is still using albuterol often at the day & wake up at night w/ SOB) add **long acting inhaled beta agonist LABA such as salmeterol or formoterol.** Using long acting beta agonist w/o inhaled steroid in asthma pts ↑ mortality (but NOT for COPD).
- **PO steroids** are a last resort

C. Steps in chronic management of COPD

1. Tiotropium or ipratropium inhaler w/ or w/o Albuterol inhaler (as monotherapy)
2. Add long acting inhaled beta agonist LABA such as salmeterol or formoterol.
3. Add inhaled steroids.
4. Add PO steroids (also consider cardiopulm rehabilitation).

For last stages, consider surgical options such as LVRS & lung transplantation.

> **Attention**: LABA can be added before inhaled steroids in asthma pts (but NOT in COPD)

Pneumococcal vaccine & annual influenza vaccine, smoking cessation (improves mortality).

D. Pneumonia Types & Management

- **Community Acquired Pneumonia (CAP):** Pneumonia acquired outside of medical facility that does NOT fit in the definition of HCAP. Standard out pt therapy is monotherapy w/ a fluoroquinolone (Levaquin) or Augmentin + Azithromycin. In hospital setting, start Ceftriaxone/Azithromycin IV.
- **Healthcare Associated Pneumonia (HCAP):** Criteria include hospitalization in acute care hospital for two or more days in last 90 days, residence in nursing home or long-term care facility in last 30 days, receiving out pt IV therapy or home wound care in last 30 days, or attending hospital clinic or dialysis center w/ in 30 days. Also included PNA that begins 48-72 hrs after hospital admission. Standard abx are Vanc & Zosyn IV (covers G+, G-, & anaerobic including MRSA &

Pseudomonas) as initial therapy. Tailor therapy according to C & S.

- **Ventilator Associated Pneumonia (VAP):** PNA occurring after 48 hrs of pt being intubated & placed on mechanical ventilation. Tx is same as for HCAP (must cover Pseudomonas).

E. Reconcile home meds

Thiss an important part of the management after MICU admission (or any hospital admission) & doing your 1st assessment/ work up along w/ initial Tx.

As a general role & due to the critical pt illness, constant ability to monitor the pt closely & the possibility of meds interactions; some meds should be held or switched to other forms.

Some examples:
- **Insulin drip** is preferred (stop PO diabetes meds in general in the hospital)
- **BP meds & diuretics** (hold in septic pts & carefully resume as BP tolerates)
- **Narcotics & pain meds** for chief complaint of AMS, HoTN or any complaints could be from the meds side effects. AMS is one of the signs of organ dysfunction & it will be clouded w/ those meds on addition of possible HoTN & respiratory failure. Restart meds as appropriate when the diagnosis is clearer & pt is responding to Tx.
- **Psychiatric & sleep meds:** antipsychotic meds like Haldol (1st generation/better in cardiac disease), olanzapine/Quetiapine (2nd generation), & benzos (same reason for holding pain meds; resume as needed). Caution w/ benzos withdrawal seizures for chronic users.
- **Some meds w/ common side effects** like diphenhydramine (for itching; anticholinergic

property causes AMS & urinary retention), Baclofen (for muscle spasm; causes AMS) **Hold meds which does NOT cause immediate benefits** like statins (if MICU admission is NOT from cardiac etiology), allopurinol, vitamins, etc (to ↓ meds interaction & ADR)

Perfusion can often be improved by administering some combination of intravenous fluids, vasopressors/ inotropic agents such as:

- **Norepinephrine (levophed):** which is strong α1 agonist (stronger than epinephrine) & β1 agonist (same as Epi)/ moderate β2 agonist (weaker than Epi). "Squeeze" good but **proarrhythmic due to β1 effect**.

> **Attention:** β2 agonist causes HoTN (receptors are in vessels) vs β1 agonist ↑ chronotropic and inotropic effect (receptors in the heart) vs α1 agonist in vessels (NOT in the heart) → vasoconstriction.

- **Phenylephrine:** which is strong α1 agonist. "Squeeze" good but do NOT affect the heart.
- **Vasopressin:** which is a V1 receptor agonist in the vascular smooth muscle of the vessels. Also "squeeze" w/o cardiac direct effect).
- **Dopamine & dobutamine:** less common
- **Epinephrine:** (β agonist mainly).

F. Constipation:

Management

- **Diet:** ↑ both total fiber & water intake. Psyllium 1 tsp daily-TID is a common 1st choice. If the pt is bed-bound & /or NOT drinking sufficient water, fiber can make the constipation worse.
- **Laxatives:** separated into 4 groups according to their mechanism of action
- **Emollients** (stool softeners): Mineral oil & docusate salts (Colace). Note: Mineral oil causes lipoid PNA if aspirated & ↓ the absorption of fat-soluble vitamins if given w/ meals.
- **Hyperosmolar agents:** Polyethylene glycol (MiraLax), lactulose, sorbitol, & glycerol. Note: Both lactulose & sorbitol are very effective & are highly recommended to use in chronic constipation if fiber & fluid supplementation alone do NOT work. Golytely is a similar laxative with some electrolytes which is indicated for bowel cleaning prior to colonoscopy
- **Saline laxatives:** Mg hydroxide (mild of magnesia) & Mg citrate (do NOT use w/ renal insufficiency because of Mg toxicity). This is usually NOT a good long-term option in the elderly.
- **Stimulant laxatives:** Castor oil, Senna (Senokot), & bisacodyl (Dulcolax). NOT recommended for long-term use. Dulcolax is a gastric irritant. Tablets are enteric coated & should NOT be broken or chewed.
- **Prokinetics:** Reglan ↑ gut motility & is sometimes used in pts on opiates. However, do NOT give it if there is concern for obstruction, as this will make it worse. Erythromycine ↑ GI motility as well.
- **Opioid induced:** Methylnaltrexone (Relistor) is indicated for the Tx of opioid-induced constipation (OIC) in pts w/ advanced illness who are receiving palliative care when response to laxative therapy

has NOT been sufficient. This is given in SQ form 8-12 mg Q daily & should be renally dosed. Naloxegol is another option.

- **Enemas:** can be used episodically for "salvage" therapy if an alternative bowel program has NOT produced a BM.

> **Attention:** Do NOT use Fleet's enemas in pts w/ renal insufficiency because of retention of phosphate (Naloxegol is another option).

- **Suppositories:** Both glycerin & bisacodyl (Dulcolax) can be used; however, they can be associated w/ cramping. They can also be used for "salvage" therapy.

G. Immune status:

Special considerations
- Most pts w/ immunodeficiency can safely receive all killed or inactivated **vaccines**. In contrast, live vaccines should NOT be given to pts w/ severe immune dysfunction.
- **Prophylactic abx** are indicated in pts w/ specific immunodeficiency disorders in order to prevent opportunistic infx: diclofenac for fungus, Bactrim for PCP infx (prophylactic dose every 48h), acyclovir.
- **PCP prophylaxis in non HIV pts:** Pts receiving a glucocorticoid dose equivalent to ≥20 mg of prednisone daily for one month or longer who also have another cause of immune-compromise; transplant pts (bone marrow or solid organs like kidney); pts receiving certain immunosuppressive drugs (purine analog or another T-cell depleting agent). Generally the need for prophylaxis is NOT

permanent; however, it depends on the indication. HIV/AIDS pts w/ T4<200 may need Bactrim until their T4 ↑

- **Neutropenic fever:** a single PO temperature of >38. 3°C (101°F) or a temperature of >38. 0°C (100. 4°F) sustained for >1 hr (NOT just subjective fever) in pts w/ absolute neutrophil count (ANB) <500. There are many etiologies for neutropenia, but some of the most common are s/p chemotherapy & acute leukemia. Cover prophylactically w/ empiric parenteral abx therapy (such as vanc/zosyn), fluconazole, & acyclovir after sending pan cultures (blood/urine/sputum), & proceed w/ the work-up as indicated (CXR & urine analysis- UA). Neutropenic fever is a medical emergency & empiric antibacterial therapy should be started w/ in 60 minutes of presentation in all pts.

Abbreviations

Term	Abbr.
Increase	↑
decrease	↓
Acute kidney injury	AKI
Alcohol	EtOH
and	&
Arterial blood gas	ABG
Atrial fibrillation	A fib
Biopsy	bx
Bone marrow	BM
Capillary blood glucose	CBG
Cardiovascular	CV
Chest pain	CP
Chest x-ray	CXR
Congestive heart failure	CHF
Coronary artery bypass surgery	CABG
Coronary artery disease	CAD
Culture	Cx
Diabetes mellitus	DM
diabetic ketoacidosis	DKA
Differential diagnosis	DDx
Dysfunction	Dysfx
Ejection fraction	EF
Electrocardiogram	EKG
End stage renal disease	ESRD

Term	Abbr.
Esophagus gastric duodenum	EGD
Headache	HA
Hemoglobin	Hgb
History	hx
Hyperosmolar hyperglycemic nonketotic syndrome	HHNS
Hypertension	HTN
Hypotension	HoTN
Herpes Zoster Virus	HZV
Infection	Infx
Intravenous	IV
Magnesium	Mg
Medical	MICU
Medication	meds
Myocardial infarction	MI
Nausea & vomiting	N/V
Nitroglycerin	NTG
Non ST elevation myocardial Infarction	NSTE MI
Oral	PO
patient	pt
Pneumonia	PNA
Pulmonary	Pulm
Reticulocyte index	RI
Serum creatinine	Cr

ST elevation myocardial Infarction	STEMI
Symptoms Sx	Sx
Treatment Tx	Tx
Urinary tract infection	UTI
Urine analysis	UA
Urine drug screen	UDS
Vacomycin	Vanc
With	w/
With out	w/o
beta blocker	B blocker
Mean artery pressure	MAP
Cardiac output	CO
Total peripheral resistance	TPR
Heart rate	HR
Stroke volume	SV
As needed	PRN
Left bundle branch block	LBBB
Right bundle branch block	RBBB
Aspirin	ASA
Gastroenterology	GI
CT angiography	CTA
Arterial blood gas	ABG
Deep venous thrombosis	DVT
Tissue Plasminogen	tPA
Jogular venous	JVD

distension	
Right ventricle	RV
Brain natriuretic peptide	BNP
Basic metabolic panel	BMP
Rapid plasma reagin	RPR
Infective endocarditis	IE
Anti nuclear antibodies	ANA
Anti-neutrophil cytoplasmic antibody	ANCA
Fecal occult blood test	FOBT
peripherally inserted central catheter	PICC line
Small bowel obstruction	SBO
Community acquired pneumonia	CAP
Healthcare acquired pneumonia	HCAP
Ventricular fibrillation	VF
Gram positive/negative	G+/-
Proton pumb inhipitor	PPI
Over the counter	OTC
Atriovenous malformation	AVM
Central nervous system	CNS
Cerebral vascular disease	CVA
Levt ventricular assist device	LVAT
Left anterior descending	LAD

Right coronary artery	RCA	Hydrochlorothiazide	HCTZ
Creatine phosphokinase	CPK	Calcium channel blocker	CCB
Patent foramen ovale	PFO	Drug adverse effect	DAE
Drug-eluting stent	DES	Pulmonary function test	PFT
partial pressure arterial oxygen	PaO2	Hemodialysis	HD
fraction of inspired oxygen	FiO2	Hemoglobin	Hgb
Acute respiratory distress syndrome	ARDS	Ventilation/perfusion	V/Q
		Esophagogastroduodenoscopy	EGD
glomerular basement membrane	GBM	Transthoracic Echocardiogram	TTE
Primary care provider	PCP	Dyspnia on exertion	DOE
Benign prostatic hyperplasia	BPH	Percutaneous coronary angiogram/intervention	PCA/ PCI
Non-invasive positive pressure ventilation	NIPPV or NIV	Obstructive sleep apenia	OSA
		Rule out	r/o
Fresh frozen plasma	FFP	Anticoagulation	Antico-agx

List of medications commonly used

Brand	(Generic) Indication
Abilify	(Aripiprazole) Antipsychotic
Actonel	(Risedronate) Osteoporosis agent
Actos	(Pioglitazone) Antidiabetic
Advair	(Fluticasone + Salmeterol) Antiasthmatic
Aldactone	(Spirinolactone) <K+ sparing diuretic>
Allegra-D	(Fexofenadine + Pseudoephedrine) Antihistamine/ Decongestant
Ambien	(Zolpidem) Hypnotic sedative
Amoxil	(Amoxicillin) Penicillin Antibiotic
Flexeril	(Cyclobenzaprine) Muscle relaxant
Aleve	(Naproxen) NSAID
Antivert	(Meclizine) Anti-vertigo agent
Aricept	(Donepezil) Antipsychotic/ Agent for Alzheimer's Dementia
Atarax	(Hydroxyzine) Antianxiety/ Antipruritic
Ativan	(Lorazepam) Antianxiety
Augmentin	(Amoxicillin/ Clavulanate) Penicillin antibiotic w/ penicillinase inhibitor
Avandia	(Rosiglitazone) Antidiabetic
Avelox	(Moxifloxacin) Fluoroquinolone antibiotic
Avodart	(Dutasteride) Prostate anti-inflammatory
Bactrim, Septra	(Sulfamethoxazole/Trimethoprim) Sulfonamide antibiotic
Bactroban	(Mupirocin) Antibacterial <topical ointment>
Benadryl	(Diphenhydramine) Antihistamine
Benicar	(Olmesartan) Antihypertensive
Bentyl	(Dicyclomine) GI antispasmotic
Boniva	(Ibandronate) Osteoporosis agent

BuSpar	(Buspirone) Antianxiety agent
Capzasin-HP	(Capsaicin cream) Arthritis pain relief
Cardizem	(Diltiazem) Antihypertensive/anginal <non-DHP CCB>
Cardura	(Doxazosin) Antihypertensive/ BPH Agent <alpha-1 antagonist>
Catapres	(Clonidine) Antihypertensive <central α2-agonist>
Ceftin	(Cefuroxime) Cephalosporin Antibiotic 2nd G
Celebrex	(Celecoxib) NSAID, selective for COX2
Celexa	(Citalopram) Antidepressant SSRI
Chantix	(Varenicline) Smoking Cessation Aid
Cialis	(Tadalafil) Erectile dysftn
Cipro	(Ciprofloxacin) Fluoroquinolone antibiotic
Cleocin	(Clindamycin) Antibiotic
Cogentin	(Benztropine Mesylate) Anti-Parkinson
Colchicine	(generic only) anti-inflammotary for gout
Combivent	(Ipratropium + Albuterol MDI) Antiasthmatic
Cordarone	(Amiodarone) Antiarrhythmic <class III>
Coreg	(Carvedilol) Antihypertensive <nonselective beta-blocker with alpha-1 blocker)
Coumadin	(Warfarin) Anticoagulant
Cozaar	(Losartan) Antihypertensive
Crestor	(Rosuvastatin) Antihyperlipidemic, high potency <HMG-CoA reductase inhibitor>
Cymbalta	(Duloxetine) Antidepressant SNRI
Deltasone	(Prednisone) Anti-inflammatory
Depakote	(Divalproex) Antiepileptic/Antipsychotic

Desyrel	(Trazadone) Antidepressant
Detrol	(Tolterodine) Urinary bladder modifier
Diflucan	(Fluconazole) Antifungal
Dilantin Kapseals	(Phenytoin) Antiepileptic
Dilaudid	(Hydromorphone) Analgesic
Diovan	(Valsartan) Antihypertensive
Ditropan	(Oxybutynin) Urinary bladder modifier
Drisdol	(Vitamin D, Ergocalciferol) Vitamin
DuoNeb	(Ipratropium + Albuterol soln) Antiasthmatic
Duragesic	(Fentanyl) Opioid Analgesic
Dyazide, Maxzide	(Triamtrene/ HCTZ) Diuretic <K+ sparing + thiazide diuretic>
Ecotrin	(Aspirin, enteric-coated) Blood Modifier <platelet inhibitor>
Effexor	(Venlafaxine) Antidepressant SNRI
Effient	(Prasurgel) antiplatelets, used similar to plavix.
Elavil	(Amitriptyline) Antidepressant TCA
Eliquis	(ApiXaban) inhibit Factor X, novel oral anticoagx
Estrace	(Estradiol) Estrogen hormone, gel/tab/patch/vaginal/IM
Evista	(Raloxifene) Osteoporosis agent
Flagyl	(Metronidazole) Antibacterial/ Antiprotozoal
Flomax	(Tamsulosin) for BPH <alpha 1-a selective blocker>
Flonase	(Fluticasone) Antiallergy
Flovent	(Fluticasone MDI) Antiasthmatic
Fosamax	(Alendronate) Osteoporosis agent
Glucophage	(Metformin) Antidiabetic
Glucotrol	(Glipizide) Antidiabetic

Glucovance	(Glyburide/ Metformin) Antidiabetic
Haldol	(Haloperidol) Antipsychotic
Humalog	(Insulin Lispro, rDNA origin) Anti-diabetic
Humulin N, Humulin R	(Regular insulin NPH, Regular insulin) Anti-diabetic
HydroDiuril	(Hydrochlorothiazide) Thiazide Diuretic
Hytrin	(Terazosin) Antihypertensive/BPH <beta-1 antagonist>
Hyzaar	(Losartan + HCT) Antihypertensive
Imdur	(Isosorbide mononitrate) Antianginal
Integrilin	(Eptifibatide), anti-platelets, used mainly in PCI. Blocks binding of fibrinogen & von Willebrand factor to glycoprotein IIb/IIIa receptor on platelet surface
Isordil	(Isosorbide dinonitrate) Antianginal
Isoptin	(Verapimil) Antihypertensive/ Antianginal
Januvia	(Sitagliptin) Antidiabetic
Keflex	(Cephalexin) Cephalosporin antibiotic
Kenalog	(Tiramcinolone Acetonide) Topical Corticosteroid
Keppra	(Levetiracetam) Anti-convulsant
Klonopin	(Clonazepam) Antiepileptic
Lamicatal	(Lamotrigine) Antiepileptic
Lanoxin	(Digoxin) Inotropic agent
Lantus	(Insulin Glargine) Anti-diabetic
Lasix	(Furosemide) Loop Diuretic
Levaquin	(Levofloxacin) Fluoroquinolone antibiotic
Lexapro	(Escitalopram) Antidepressant SSRI
Lioresal	(Baclofen) Muscle relaxant
Lipitor	(Atorvastatin) Antihyperlipidemic, high potency <HMG-CoA reductase

inhibitor>

Lopid	(Gemfibrozil) Antihyperlipidemic <activate PPARa>
Lopressor	(Metoprolol Tartrate) Antihypertensive < B blocker>
Lortab, Vicodin	(Hydrocodone w/ tylenol) Opioid Analgesic
Lotensin	(Benazepril) Antihypertensive <ACE Inhibitor>
Lotrisone	(Clotrimazole w/ Betamethasone) Topical Antifungal
Lovaza	(Omega-3 FAs) Antihyperlipidemic
Lyrica	(Pregabalin) Anti-convulsant/Antineuralgic
Macrodantin, Macrobid	(Nitrofurantoin) Antibacterial
Medrol	(Methylpredisolone) Anti-inflammatory
Methadose, Dolophine	(Methadone) Opioid Analgesic
Micronase	(Glyburide) Antidiabetic
Miralax	(Polyethylene Glycol 2250) Laxative
Mobic	(Meloxicam) NSAID, non-selective COX inhipitor
Motrin	(Ibuprofen) NSAID
MS Contin	(Morphine Sulfate) Opioid Analgesic, long acting
Mytussin AC, Robutussin AC	(Codeine Phosphate w/ Guaifenesin) Antitussive/Expectorant
Namenda	(Memantine) Agent for Alzheimer's Dementia
Nasacort AQ	(Triamcinolone) Antiallergy
Nasonex	(Mometasone) Antiallergy
Neurontin	(Gabapentin) Antiepileptic, for neuropathy as well.
Nexium	(Esomeprazole) PPI

Niaspan	(Niacin) Antihyperlipidemic <increase lipoprotein lipase activity>
Nitrostat	(Nitroglycerin) Antianginal
Nizoral	(Ketoconazole) Antifungal
Norvasc	(Amlopidine) Antihypertensive <DHP CCB>
Novolog	(Insulin Aspart, rDNA origin) Anti-diabetic
NuvaRing	(Etonogestrel & Ethinyl estradiol) Contraceptive
Nystop	(Nystatin) Antifungal Antibiotic
Omnicef	(Cefdinir) Cephalosporin antibiotic, PO 3rd G
Oraped	(Prednisolone) Anti-inflammatory
Othro-Cyclen, Sprintec	(Norgestimate & Ethinyl estradiol) Oral contraceptive
Ovral, Lo/Ovral, Ogestrel,	(Noregestrel & Ethinyl estradiol) Oral contraceptive
Oxycontin	(Oxycodone CR) Opioid Analgesic
OxyIR, Roxicodone	(Oxycodone IR) Opioid Analgesic
Pamelor	(Nortriptyline) Antidepressant TCA
Paxil	(Paroxetine) Antidepressant SSRI
Pepcid	(Famotadine) Anti-ulcer agent
Percocet	(Oxycodone w/ tylenol) Opioid Analgesic
Phenergan	(Promethazine) Anti-emetic
Plaquenil	(Hydroxychloroquine) Antimalarial
Plavix	(Clopidogrel) Platelet Inhibitor
Pradaxa	(Dabigatran) inhibit thrombin, novel anticoagx
Pravachol	(Pravastatin) Antihyperlipidemic <HMG-CoA reductase inhibitor>
Premarin	(Conjugated estrogens) Estrogen

	Hormone
Prilosec	(Omeprazole) Anti-ulcer agent
Procardia, Nifedical, Adalet	(Nifedipine) Antihypertensive/ Antianginal <DHP CCB>
Proscar	(Finasteride) Prostate anti-inflammatory
Protonix	(Pantoprazole) Anti-ulcer agent
Proventil, Ventolin, Proair	(Albuterol) Anti-asthmatic
Prozac	(Fluoxetine) Antidepressant SSRI
Pyridium	(Phenazopyridine) Urinary tract analgesic
Ranexa	(Ranolazine) 2nd line anti-anginal, unknown mechanism.
Reglan	(Metoclopramide) Anti-emetic
Remeron	(Mirtazapine) Antidepressant
Requip	(Ropinirole) Anti-Parkinson, restless leg syndrome
Risperdal	(Risperidone) Antipsychotic
Robaxin	(Methocarbamol) Muscle relaxant
Seroquel	(Quetiapine) Antipsychotic
Singulair	(Montelukast) Antiasthmatic
Soma	(Carisoprodol) Muscle relaxant
Spiriva	(Tiotropium) Antiasthmatic
Suboxone	(Buprenorphine w/ Naloxone) Agent for Opioid Dependence
Synthroid, Levothyroid	(Levothyroxine) Thyroid hormone
Tamiflu	(Oseltamivir) Antiviral
Temovate	(Clobetasol Proprionate) Topical Anti-inflammatory
Tessalon	(Benzonatate) Antitussive
Topamax	(Topiramate) Antiepileptic

Toprol-XL	(Metoprolol Succinate) Antihypertensive <selective beta-1 blocker>
Tricor	(Fenofibrate) Antihyperlipidemic (mainly TG)
Tussionex	(Clorpheniramine w/ Hydrocodone) Antitussive
Ultram, Ryzolt	(Tramadol HCl) Analgesic
Valium	(Diazepam) Antianxiety
Valtrex	(Valacyclovir) Antiviral
Veramyst	(Fluticasone) Antiallergy
Viagra	(Sildenafil) Erectile dysftn
Victosa	(Liraglutide) SQ meds for DMII & obesity, increase insulin
Vibramycin	(Doxycycline) Tetracycline antibiotic
Avelox	(Moxifloxacin) Fluoroquinolone antibiotic
Vivelle-Dot	(Estradiol) Hormonal replacement <topical>
Voltaren	(Diclofenac) NSAID
Wellbutrin	(Bupropion) Antidepressant
Xanax	(Alprazolam) Antianxiety
Xarelto	(RivaroXaban) inhibit Factor X, novel oral anticoagx.
Xopenex	(Levalbuterol) Antiasthmatic
Yasmin, Ocella	(Drospirenone & Ethinyl estradiol) Oral contraceptive
Zanaflex	(Tizanidine) Muscle relaxant
Zantac	(Ranitidine) Anti-ulcer agent
Zebeta	(Bisoprolol) Antihypertensive
Zestril	(Lisinopril) Antihypertensive <ACE Inhibitor>
Zetia	(Ezetimibe) Antihyperlipidemic <inhibits intestinal absorption of cholesterol>

Zithromax, Z pack	(Azithromycin) Macrolide Antibiotic
Zocor	(Simvastatin) Antihyperlipidemic <HMG-CoA reductase inhibitor>
Zoloft	(Sertraline) Antidepressant SSRI
Zosyn	(Piperacillin/tazobactam) Antibiotic
Zovirax	(Acyclovir) Antiviral
Zyloprim	(Allopurinol) Agent for gout
Zyprexa	(Olanzapine) Atypical Antipsychotic

References

1. Harrison's Principles of Internal Medicine, 18th edition. Dan L. Longo, Editor, Anthony S. Fauci, Editor, Dennis L. Kasper, Editor, Stephen L. Hauser, Editor, J. Larry Jameson, Editor, Joseph Loscalzo, Editor
2. Foster C, Misry NF, Peddi PF, Sharma S. The Washington Manual of Medical Therapeutics. 33rd edition. Department of Medicine, Washington University School of Medicine. Wolters Kluwer/Lippincott Williams & Wilkins; 2010.
3. Sabatine MS. Pocket Medicine (The Massachusetts General Hospital Handbook of Internal Medicine). Fourth Edition. Wolters Kluwer/Lippincott Williams & Wilkins; 2010.
4. Rodvold KA, McConeghy KW et al. Methicillin-Resistant Staphylococcus aureus Therapy: Past, Present, and Future. CID;2014(1):S20-27.
5. Foster C, Misry NF, Peddi PF, Sharma S. The Washington Manual of Medical Therapeutics. 33rd edition. Department of Medicine, Washington University School of Medicine. Wolters Kluwer/Lippincott Williams & Wilkins; 2010.
6. Surawicz CM, Brandt LJ, Binion DG et al. Guidelines for Diagnosis, Treatment, and Prevention of Clostridium difficile infections. The American Journal of Gastroenterology. 2013;108(4):478-498.
7. Momeni M, Crucitti M, De Kock M. Patient-controlled analgesia in the management of postoperative pain. Drugs. 2006;66(18):2321-37.
8. Sabatine MS. Pocket Medicine (The Massachusetts General Hospital Handbook of Internal Medicine). Fourth Edition. Wolters Kluwer/Lippincott Williams & Wilkins; 2010.
9. Birdwell BG, Herbers JE, Kroenke K. Evaluating chest pain. The patient's presentation style alters the physician's diagnostic approach. Arch Intern Med 1993; 153:1991.
10. Pavlik VN, Hyman DJ, Wendt JA, Orengo C. Association of a culturally defined syndrome (nervios) with chest pain and DSM-IV affective disorders in Hispanic patients referred for cardiac stress testing. Ethn Dis 2004; 14:505.
11. Challenging existing paradigms in ischemic heart disease: the NHBLI-sponsored women's ischemia syndrome evaluation (WISE). J Am Coll Cardiol 2006; 47:1S.
12. D'Antono B, Dupuis G, Fortin C, et al. Angina symptoms in men and women with stable coronary artery disease and evidence of exercise-induced myocardial perfusion defects. Am Heart J 2006; 151:813.
13. von Kodolitsch Y, Schwartz AG, Nienaber CA. Clinical prediction of acute aortic dissection. Arch Intern Med 2000; 160:2977.
14. McGee, S. Pulmonary embolism. In: Evidence based physical diagnosis, 2, Saunders Elsevier, 2007. p.365.

15. Marcus GM, Cohen J, Varosy PD, et al. The utility of gestures in patients with chest discomfort. Am J Med 2007; 120:83.
16. Davies HA, Jones DB, Rhodes J, Newcombe RG. Angina-like esophageal pain: differentiation from cardiac pain by history. J Clin Gastroenterol 1985; 7:477. DWORKEN HJ, BIEL FJ, MACHELLA TE. Supradiaphragmatic reference of pain from the colon. Gastroenterology 1952; 22:222.
17. Ryle JA. Visceral pain and referred pain. Lancet 1926; 1:895.
18. Selzer M, Spencer WA. Convergence of visceral and cutaneous afferent pathways in the lumbar spinal cord. Brain Res 1969; 14:331.
19. Purcell TB. Nonsurgical and extraperitoneal causes of abdominal pain. Emerg Med Clin North Am 1989; 7:721.
20. Saik RP, Greenburg AG, Farris JM, Peskin GW. Spectrum of cholangitis. Am J Surg 1975; 130:143.
21. Go VL, Everhart JE. Pancreatitis. In: Digestive diseases in the United States: Epidemiology and impact, Everhart JE (Ed), National Institutes of Health, National Institute of Diabetes and Digestive and Kidney Diseases. US Government Printing Office, Washington, DC 1994. p.693.
22. Talley NJ, Colin-Jones D, Koch KL, et al. Functional dyspepsia: A classification with guidelines for diagnosis and management. Gastroenterol Int 1992; 4:145.
23. Flanagin BA, Mitchell MT, Thistlethwaite WA, Alverdy JC. Diagnosis and treatment of atypical presentations of hiatal hernia following bariatric surgery. Obes Surg 2010; 20:386.
24. Beeson MS. Splenic infarct presenting as acute abdominal pain in an older patient. J Emerg Med 1996; 14:319.
25. Nores M, Phillips EH, Morgenstern L, Hiatt JR. The clinical spectrum of splenic infarction. Am Surg 1998; 64:182.
26. Franklin QJ, Compeggie M. Splenic syndrome in sickle cell trait: four case presentations and a review of the literature. Mil Med 1999; 164:230.
27. Görg C, Seifart U, Görg K. Acute, complete splenic infarction in cancer patient is associated with a fatal outcome. Abdom Imaging 2004; 29:224. Hung JJ, Hsu HS, Huang CS, Yang KY. Tracheoesophageal fistula and tracheo-subclavian artery fistula after tracheostomy. Eur J Cardiothorac Surg 2007; 32:676.
28. Komatsu T, Sowa T, Fujinaga T, et al. Tracheo-innominate artery fistula: two case reports and a clinical review. Ann Thorac Cardiovasc Surg 2013; 19:60.
29. Choudhary C, Bandyopadhyay D, Salman R, et al. Broncho-vascular fistulas from self-expanding metallic stents: A retrospective case review. Ann Thorac Med 2013; 8:116.
30. Savale L, Parrot A, Khalil A, et al. Cryptogenic hemoptysis: from a benign to a life-threatening pathologic vascular condition. Am J Respir Crit Care Med 2007; 175:1181.

31. Kuzucu A, Gürses I, Soysal O, et al. Dieulafoy's disease: a cause of massive hemoptysis that is probably underdiagnosed. Ann Thorac Surg 2005; 80:1126.
32. Kolb T, Gilbert C, Fishman EK, et al. Dieulafoy's disease of the bronchus. Am J Respir Crit Care Med 2012; 186:1191.
33. Muniappan A, Tapias LF, Butala P, et al. Surgical therapy of pulmonary aspergillomas: a 30-year North American experience. Ann Thorac Surg 2014; 97:432.
34. Farid S, Mohamed S, Devbhandari M, et al. Results of surgery for chronic pulmonary Aspergillosis, optimal antifungal therapy and proposed high risk factors for recurrence--a National Centre's experience. J Cardiothorac Surg 2013; 8:180.
35. Ahmed S, Mohammad WW, Hamid F, et al. The 2011 dengue haemorrhagic fever outbreak in Lahore - an account of clinical parameters and pattern of haemorrhagic complications. J Coll Physicians Surg Pak 2013; 23:463.
36. Sareli AE, Janssen WJ, Sterman D, et al. Clinical problem-solving. What's the connection? - A 26-year-old white man presented to our referral hospital with a 1-month history of persistent cough productive of white sputum, which was occasionally tinged with blood. N Engl J Med 2008; 358:626.
37. Drent M, Wessels S, Jacobs JA, Thijssen H. Association of diffuse alveolar haemorrhage with acquired vitamin K deficiency. Respiration 2000; 67:697.
38. Ikeda M, Tanaka H, Sadamatsu K. Diffuse alveolar hemorrhage as a complication of dual antiplatelet therapy for acute coronary syndrome. Cardiovasc Revasc Med 2011; 12:407.
39. Chen BC, Sheth NR, Dadzie KA, et al. Hemodialysis for the treatment of pulmonary hemorrhage from dabigatran overdose. Am J Kidney Dis 2013; 62:591.
40. Heck SL, Blom P, Berstad A. Accuracy and complications in computed tomography fluoroscopy-guided needle biopsies of lung masses. Eur Radiol 2006; 16:1387.
41. Choi JW, Park CM, Goo JM, et al. C-arm cone-beam CT-guided percutaneous transthoracic needle biopsy of small (≤ 20 mm) lung nodules: diagnostic accuracy and complications in 161 patients. AJR Am J Roentgenol 2012; 199:W322.
42. Lee SM, Park CM, Lee KH, et al. C-arm cone-beam CT-guided percutaneous transthoracic needle biopsy of lung nodules: clinical experience in 1108 patients. Radiology 2014; 271:291.
43. Augoulea A, Lambrinoudaki I, Christodoulakos G. Thoracic endometriosis syndrome. Respiration 2008; 75:113.
44. Sandler A, Gray R, Perry MC, et al. Paclitaxel-carboplatin alone or with bevacizumab for non-small-cell lung cancer. N Engl J Med 2006; 355:2542.

45. Cho YJ, Murgu SD, Colt HG. Bronchoscopy for bevacizumab-related hemoptysis. Lung Cancer 2007; 56:465.
46. Karlson-Stiber C, Höjer J, Sjöholm A, et al. Nitrogen dioxide pneumonitis in ice hockey players. J Intern Med 1996; 239:451.
47. Centers for Disease Control and Prevention (CDC). Exposure to nitrogen dioxide in an indoor ice arena - New Hampshire, 2011. MMWR Morb Mortal Wkly Rep 2012; 61:139. American College of Cardiology Foundation, American Heart Association, European Society of Cardiology, et al. Management of patients with atrial fibrillation (compilation of 2006 ACCF/AHA/ESC and 2011 ACCF/AHA/HRS recommendations): a report of the American College of Cardiology/American Heart Association Task Force on practice guidelines. Circulation 2013; 127:1916.
48. January CT, Wann LS, Alpert JS, et al. 2014 AHA/ACC/HRS guideline for the management of patients with atrial fibrillation: a report of the American College of Cardiology/American Heart Association Task Force on practice guidelines and the Heart Rhythm Society. Circulation 2014; 130:e199.
49. January CT, Wann LS, Alpert JS, et al. 2014 AHA/ACC/HRS guideline for the management of patients with atrial fibrillation: executive summary: a report of the American College of Cardiology/American Heart Association Task Force on practice guidelines and the Heart Rhythm Society. Circulation 2014; 130:2071.
50. Wyse DG, Van Gelder IC, Ellinor PT, et al. Lone atrial fibrillation: does it exist? J Am Coll Cardiol 2014; 63:1715.
51. Kopecky SL, Gersh BJ, McGoon MD, et al. The natural history of lone atrial fibrillation. A population-based study over three decades. N Engl J Med 1987; 317:669.
52. Brand FN, Abbott RD, Kannel WB, Wolf PA. Characteristics and prognosis of lone atrial fibrillation. 30-year follow-up in the Framingham Study. JAMA 1985; 254:3449.
53. Kannel WB, Abbott RD, Savage DD, McNamara PM. Epidemiologic features of chronic atrial fibrillation: the Framingham study. N Engl J Med 1982; 306:1018.
54. Lévy S, Maarek M, Coumel P, et al. Characterization of different subsets of atrial fibrillation in general practice in France: the ALFA study. The College of French Cardiologists. Circulation 1999; 99:3028.
55. Takahashi N, Seki A, Imataka K, Fujii J. Clinical features of paroxysmal atrial fibrillation. An observation of 94 patients. Jpn Heart J 1981; 22:143.
56. Clemency J, Dulhoste MN, Laiter C, et al. Flecainide acetate in the prevention of paroxysmal atrial fibrillation: a nine-

month follow-up of more than 500 patients. Am J Cardiol 1992; 70:44A.
57. EVANS W, SWANN P. Lone auricular fibrillation. Br Heart J 1954; 16:189.
58. LAMB LE, POLLARD LW. ATRIAL FIBRILLATION IN FLYING PERSONNEL. Circulation 1964; 29:694.
59. Peter RH, Gracey JG, Beach TB. A clinical profile of idiopathic atrial fibrillation. A functional disorder of atrial rhythm. Ann Intern Med 1968; 68:1288.
60. Rostagno C, Bacci F, Martelli M, et al. Clinical course of lone atrial fibrillation since first symptomatic arrhythmic episode. Am J Cardiol 1995; 76:837. Sterns RH, Silver SM. Salt and water: read the package insert. QJM 2003; 96:549.
61. Rose BD, Post TW. Clinical Physiology of Acid-Base and Electrolyte Disorders, 5th ed, McGraw-Hill, New York 2001. p.441.
62. Lu KC, Hsu YJ, Chiu JS, et al. Effects of potassium supplementation on the recovery of thyrotoxic periodic paralysis. Am J Emerg Med 2004; 22:544.
63. McCowen KC, Malhotra A, Bistrian BR. Stress-induced hyperglycemia. Crit Care Clin 2001; 17:107. tension. J Appl Physiol Respir Environ Exerc Physiol 1984; 57:686.
64. Taguchi O, Kikuchi Y, Hida W, et al. Effects of bronchoconstriction and external resistive loading on the sensation of dyspnea. J Appl Physiol (1985) 1991; 71:2183.
65. Moy ML, Woodrow Weiss J, Sparrow D, et al. Quality of dyspnea in bronchoconstriction differs from external resistive loads. Am J Respir Crit Care Med 2000; 162:451.
66. Clark AL, Piepoli M, Coats AJ. Skeletal muscle and the control of ventilation on exercise: evidence for metabolic receptors. Eur J Clin Invest 1995; 25:299.
67. Clark A, Volterrani M, Swan JW, et al. Leg blood flow, metabolism and exercise capacity in chronic stable heart failure. Int J Cardiol 1996; 55:127.
68. Killian KJ, Leblanc P, Martin DH, et al. Exercise capacity and ventilatory, circulatory, and symptom limitation in patients with chronic airflow limitation. Am Rev Respir Dis 1992; 146:935.
69. Melzack R, Torgerson WS. On the language of pain. Anesthesiology 1971; 34:50.
70. Melzack R. The McGill Pain Questionnaire: major properties and scoring methods. Pain 1975; 1:277.
71. Hunter M, Philips C. The experience of headache pain--an assessment of the qualities of tension headache pain. Pain 1981; 10:209. Netea MG, Kullberg BJ, Van der Meer JW. Circulating cytokines as mediators of fever. Clin Infect Dis 2000; 31 Suppl 5:S178.
72. Blatteis CM, Sehic E, Li S. Pyrogen sensing and signaling: old views and new concepts. Clin Infect Dis 2000; 31 Suppl 5:S168.

73. Saper CB, Breder CD. The neurologic basis of fever. N Engl J Med 1994; 330:1880.
74. Mitchell, JD, Grocott, HP, Phillips-Bute, B, et al. Cytokine secretion after cardiac surgery and its relationship to postoperative fever. Cytokine 2007; 39:37.
75. Dauleh MI, Rahman S, Townell NH. Open versus laparoscopic cholecystectomy: a comparison of postoperative temperature. J R Coll Surg Edinb 1995; 40:116.
76. Clark JA, Bar-Yosef S, Anderson A, et al. Postoperative hyperthermia following off-pump versus on-pump coronary artery bypass surgery. J Cardiothorac Vasc Anesth 2005; 19:426.
77. Ghert M, Allen B, Davids J, et al. Increased postoperative febrile response in children with osteogenesis imperfecta. J Pediatr Orthop 2003; 23:261. Rocha-Singh KJ, Eisenhauer AC, Textor SC, et al. Atherosclerotic Peripheral Vascular Disease Symposium II: intervention for renal artery disease. Circulation 2008; 118:2873.
78. Bortman G, Sellanes M, Odell DS, et al. Discrepancy between pre- and post-transplant diagnosis of end-stage dilated cardiomyopathy. Am J Cardiol 1994; 74:921.
79. Marwick TH. The viable myocardium: epidemiology, detection, and clinical implications. Lancet 1998; 351:815.
80. Allman KC, Shaw LJ, Hachamovitch R, Udelson JE. Myocardial viability testing and impact of revascularization on prognosis in patients with coronary artery disease and left ventricular dysfunction: a meta-analysis. J Am Coll Cardiol 2002; 39:1151.
81. Repetto A, Dal Bello B, Pasotti M, et al. Coronary atherosclerosis in end-stage idiopathic dilated cardiomyopathy: an innocent bystander? Eur Heart J 2005; 26:1519.
82. Jessup M, Brozena S. Heart failure. N Engl J Med 2003; 348:2007.
83. Koelling TM, Aaronson KD, Cody RJ, et al. Prognostic significance of mitral regurgitation and tricuspid regurgitation in patients with left ventricular systolic dysfunction. Am Heart J 2002; 144:524.
84. Fonarow GC, Yancy CW, Hernandez AF, et al. Potential impact of optimal implementation of evidence-based heart failure therapies on mortality. Am Heart J 2011; 161:1024.
85. Willenheimer R, van Veldhuisen DJ, Silke B, et al. Effect on survival and hospitalization of initiating treatment for chronic heart failure with bisoprolol followed by enalapril, as compared with the opposite sequence: results of the randomized Cardiac Insufficiency Bisoprolol Study (CIBIS) III. Circulation 2005; 112:2426.
86. Sliwa K, Norton GR, Kone N, et al. Impact of initiating carvedilol before angiotensin-converting enzyme inhibitor

therapy on cardiac function in newly diagnosed heart failure. J Am Coll Cardiol 2004; 44:1825.
87. Fang JC. Angiotensin-converting enzyme inhibitors or beta-blockers in heart failure: does it matter who goes first? Circulation 2005; 112:2380.
88. Bristow MR, Gilbert EM, Abraham WT, et al. Carvedilol produces dose-related improvements in left ventricular function and survival in subjects with chronic heart failure. MOCHA Investigators. Circulation 1996; 94:2807.
89. Wikstrand J, Hjalmarson A, Waagstein F, et al. Dose of metoprolol CR/XL and clinical outcomes in patients with heart failure: analysis of the experience in metoprolol CR/XL randomized intervention trial in chronic heart failure (MERIT-HF). J Am Coll Cardiol 2002; 40:491.
90. Faris R, Flather MD, Purcell H, et al. Diuretics for heart failure. Cochrane Database Syst Rev 2006; :CD003838.
91. Effect of enalapril on mortality and the development of heart failure in asymptomatic patients with reduced left ventricular ejection fractions. The SOLVD Investigattors. N Engl J Med 1992; 327:685.
92. Cohn JN, Johnson G, Ziesche S, et al. A comparison of enalapril with hydralazine-isosorbide dinitrate in the treatment of chronic congestive heart failure. N Engl J Med 1991; 325:303.
93. Effects of enalapril on mortality in severe congestive heart failure. Results of the Cooperative North Scandinavian Enalapril Survival Study (CONSENSUS). The CONSENSUS Trial Study Group. N Engl J Med 1987; 316:1429.
94. Effect of enalapril on survival in patients with reduced left ventricular ejection fractions and congestive heart failure. The SOLVD Investigators. N Engl J Med 1991; 325:293.
95. Flather MD, Yusuf S, Køber L, et al. Long-term ACE-inhibitor therapy in patients with heart failure or left-ventricular dysfunction: a systematic overview of data from individual patients. ACE-Inhibitor Myocardial Infarction Collaborative Group. Lancet 2000; 355:1575.
96. Kostis JB, Shelton BJ, Yusuf S, et al. Tolerability of enalapril initiation by patients with left ventricular dysfunction: results of the medication challenge phase of the Studies of Left Ventricular Dysfunction. Am Heart J 1994; 128:358.
97. Packer M, Poole-Wilson PA, Armstrong PW, et al. Comparative effects of low and high doses of the angiotensin-converting enzyme inhibitor, lisinopril, on morbidity and mortality in chronic heart failure. ATLAS Study Group. Circulation 1999; 100:2312.
98. Delahaye F, de Gevigney G. Is the optimal dose of angiotensin-converting enzyme inhibitors in patients with congestive heart failure definitely established? J Am Coll Cardiol 2000; 36:2096.

99. Brophy JM, Joseph L, Rouleau JL. Beta-blockers in congestive heart failure. A Bayesian meta-analysis. Ann Intern Med 2001; 134:550.
100. Effect of metoprolol CR/XL in chronic heart failure: Metoprolol CR/XL Randomised Intervention Trial in Congestive Heart Failure (MERIT-HF). Lancet 1999; 353:2001. Ahmed A, Rich MW, Fleg JL, et al. Effects of digoxin on morbidity and mortality in diastolic heart failure: the ancillary digitalis investigation group trial. Circulation 2006; 114:397.